The Connection Formula

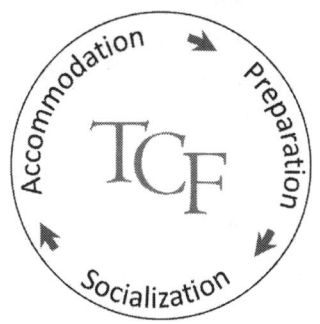

How to *Autism-ize* Your Thinking *and* Become Your Child's Lifeline

Nancy Swanberg

Connection Formula Resources, LLC
www.connectionformula.com

The Connection Formula:
How to Autism-ize Your Thinking and Become Your Child's Lifeline

Copyright © 2014 Nancy Swanberg
All rights reserved.

This book is based on the experiences of the author, and is intended to provide information about the author's viewpoint and methodologies. This book does not constitute a substitute for professional psychological treatment, therapy, or other types of professional advice and intervention; nor is it specific to any individual's situation or needs. The reader should therefore use common sense when adapting and applying the advice in this book, and consult the appropriate professionals with any and all questions, concerns, or special circumstances regarding children in the reader's care. The author and publisher have made every effort to assure accuracy and clarity, and do not assume and hereby disclaim any liability to any party for any loss, damage or disruption caused by misinterpretation or inappropriate application of the information herein, whether due to content errors, omissions, typographical or grammatical mistakes or any other cause.

Publisher's Cataloging-In-Publication Data
(Prepared by The Donohue Group, Inc.)

Swanberg, Nancy.
   The connection formula : how to autism-ize your thinking and become your child's lifeline / Nancy Swanberg.

   pages : illustrations ; cm

   ISBN-13: 978-0-692-33473-7
   ISBN-10: 0-692-33473-4

   1. Autistic children--Life skills guides. 2. Autistic children--Education. 3. Social skills in children. 4. Parent and child. I. Title.

HQ773.8 S93 2014
649/.154   2014921004

First Edition
Cover photo by Laurel Grondin

Connection Formula Resources, LLC • Worcester, Massachusetts

In memory of my mom, Anne Goulding, who always knew the secret of unconditional love.

Acknowledgements

First, a special thanks to all the members, past and present, of the Student-to-Student Autism Connection. You have inspired many people to understand and care more deeply about autism. I am one of them.

To every Autistic person I have known: thank you for teaching me the power of new perspectives.

To all who have believed in this book and offered encouragement and advice: it has been a very long journey. I am grateful for your patience!

Author's Note

In this book I will generally use identity-first language ("Autistic child") over person-first language ("child with autism"). Many Autistic self-advocates have made it clear that this is their preference. Those I've had the pleasure to work with are proud to be Autistic. They do not see autism as something negative, and I wholeheartedly support their viewpoint.

Contents

Preface xv
About This Book xvii
   Who This Book Is About xviii
   Who This Book Is For xix

Introduction
Safe and Understood

1. Worlds Apart 23
   My Perspective 25
   Four Core Principles 26

2. The Compassion Gap 33
   What Is Social Information? 35
   What Is a Social Learning Disability? 37
   Get to Know Your Child's World 39

3. What Is the Connection Formula? 43
   Socialization 3-2-1 44
   Part 1: Accommodation 45
   Part 2: Preparation 47
   Part 3: Socialization 48
   The Essential First Step 50
   Aim for the Possible 51

Part 1: Accommodation
Making Life Accessible

4. Watch Your Language 55
    Be Careful with Idioms 56
    Avoid Sarcasm 60
    Mark Up Your Language with Gestures 61
    Abbreviate Your Language 63
    Using Metaphors to Connect 65
    Language in Perspective 65

5. Enter the Confusion Detective 69

6. Facts Before Feelings 73
    The Running Commentary Technique 74
    Comments Before Questions 77
    Give Concrete Choices 79
    Keep the Conversation Going 80
    "I don't know" Is an Okay Answer 81
    The True or False Game 83
    Feeling Phrases 86
    Find Connecting Logic 89
    Basics Before Social Skills 91

7. A Child's Lifeline 95
    Fear of Feelings 95
    Looking for a Superhero 96

8. Make Problems Visible 99
    Visual 1-5 Scales 100
    The Safety Scale 101
    The Logic Scale 102
    The Feeling Scale 103

Introducing the Scales to Your Child 104
Problem Scale Variations 104
The Problem Pyramid 105
Checking Your Work 105

9. Change Is a Nightmare 107
Trauma and Loss 107
The Disappointment Ratio 108
Recalibrate Your Compassion Meter 109

10. Make Life Predictable 111
Sequencing Life with Visual Schedules 111
Making Routines Concrete 114
Introducing the Idea 115
The Sequential Walkthrough 117
Sequencing with Rating Scales 121

Part 2: Preparation

Connect Before Correct

11. Conceptual Readiness 127
What Is a Concept Gap? 127
Imitation Without Understanding 129
Unexpected Priorities 130
Everything Can't Happen at Once 131
Life Is Illogical 132
Disconnected Social Norms 133
Context Is Everything 134
Where Are the Anchor Points? 137
Behavior for No Reason 137
Neurotypical Blind Spots 138

12. Emotional Readiness 143

    Behaviors Reveal a Child's Emotional State 144
    "Connect Before Correct" Moments 146
    Aligning Your Frame of Reference 148
    Think *What If* 149
    Know Your Impact 150
    Begin the Connection Process 152
    Leading the Behavior 153
    Reprogramming Your Responses 155

13. Own the Misunderstanding 159
    Did Anyone Ever Tell You 160
    About Change and Surprises 161
    About Idioms 162
    About Fairness 163
    About Compliments 163
    About Rudeness 164
    About Mistakes 166
    About Logic 167
    A Measure of Safety 169

14. A Concept Gap Journey 171

15. Unconfusing the Rules 179
    The Tangle of Exceptions 180
    The Logic of Rules 183
    The "What's the Bigger Problem" Game 184
    Very Important Information! 186
    Correcting the Backstory 188
    Rules, Laws and Guidelines 189
    Agreements, Negotiations and Promises 190
    Child-Empowering Rules 191

16. Problem Solving 195

First Connect 196
Getting the Problem on the Table 199
Minimize Stress 203
Make a Plan to Make a Plan 204
Be Specific and Concrete 205
Validate, Explain, Arrange 206
The Problem Jar 210
Parent Request Forms 211
A Plan Is a Promise 212
Creating a "Bad Surprise" Plan 214
Bad Surprise Tokens 216
Transitions and Waiting Activities 216
Tips for Problem Solving 219

17. Social Readiness 221
The Paradox Problem 222

Part 3: Socialization

Creating Shared Moments

18. Shared Moments 229
Proving the Value of the Moment 230
Yielding Your End of the Moment 231
The Friendship Experience 232
What Is Social Relatedness? 234

19. Job Description for a Social Coach 239

20. Family Fun Time 243
Setting Up the Idea 244
Organizing the Environment 245
Organizing the Schedule 247
Preparing the Activities 248

- False Starts and Big Discoveries ... 250
- Transitioning In ... 251
- Keeping Things Moving ... 251
- Making Everything Fun ... 252
- Letting It Be One-Sided ... 253
- Taking Turns ... 253
- Winning and Losing ... 255
- Make Encouraging Comments ... 257
- Handling Criticism ... 258
- Handling Interruptions ... 259
- Watching and Guiding ... 260
- Relaxing the Structure ... 262
- Seeing Through Chaos ... 262
- Transitioning Out ... 264
- Groundwork for Play Dates ... 266

21. Social Choreography ... 267
- Thinking in Details ... 268
- Why Are We Doing This? ... 269
- What Will You Do If...? ... 270
- When Do I Do Something? ... 273

22. Components of Social Independence ... 277
- Valid Reporting ... 279
- Accepting Feedback ... 286
- Self-Observation ... 288
- Effective Self-Advocacy ... 289
- Independent Social Learning ... 291
- Seeing the Pain ... 294

23. Planning a Successful Play Date ... 299
- Who Does the Planning? ... 300
- What Are Your Child's Needs? ... 301

Contents

Friendship Matching 303
Building the Concept 305
Preparing Your Child for the Play Date 307
During the Play Date 309
The Schedule 310
Let Fun Bubble to the Top 311

24. Safe Passage 313

Preface

Autistic children misunderstand the world, and the world misunderstands them. The misunderstandings are continuous, profound, and systematically overlooked. As a psychotherapist, I have seen the consequences firsthand. All too frequently these children suffer from anxiety, depression, and even thoughts of suicide. It's time to think about a system that looks at the whole child and heads off these concerns with a proactive and consistent plan.

Emotional problems in Autistic children often go undetected and untreated because, frankly, the autism gets all the attention. Serious issues fall by the wayside, and are sometimes made worse by well-meaning professionals who are fooled by appearances and focus mainly on behavior. A child is frightened and confused in a baffling world, yet some widely accepted practices do not even consider their feelings. Children on the autism spectrum can feel bullied and abused by the very people they would look to for help due to the failure of so many to understand the child's viewpoint. And so the gulf of understanding is compounded by another gulf. I call it a *compassion gap*.

Whose job is it to remedy this situation? Certainly not the child's! We as adults are supposed to have the right answers, but precious few among us seem to recognize the extent to which outer impressions can be out of sync with an Autistic child's inner experience. Before you can be a child's lifeline, you will have to go through the looking-glass to a world that is very different from your own.

Are you willing?

People tend to offer the help they know how to give, not the help that is actually needed. Learning the difference is a quite a journey. It starts by accommodating the child, seeing things from their perspective in order to establish an authentic connection. Above all, you will need to help the child feel safe and understood. That is the essence of The Connection Formula. Is it an instant answer? No, not at all. Is it even really a "formula?" I'll put it this way: neurotypical thinking about autism is itself a formula, an oversimplified one that is often counter-productive. I am offering a way to reformulate your approach – to *autism-ize* your thinking, so to speak. It's time to replace outdated assumptions with a framework for expanding our awareness of what life is like for children on the spectrum. With a greater depth of understanding we can offer a broader range of help.

This book explains what you can do right now to make an Autistic child's life a little easier for them to navigate, and gives you tools to build with, day by day. I hope you'll catch and embrace these ideas. My goal is to help you nurture the connection with the Autistic children in your life. I guarantee they crave that connection, even if all evidence says otherwise. It's very easy to be fooled by appearances. Don't worry; we're going to work on that.

Some people have already begun to autism-ize their viewpoint. For you I offer a cohesive system to help organize your approach and deepen your insights. Understandably, many others find it difficult to shift their way of thinking about autism. Those who sincerely try will gain more compassion for the difficulties faced by Autistic children when the world asks them to shift *their* way of thinking. The more people who make an effort to close the compassion gap, the less stressful life will be for children on the autism spectrum.

We can do better. Let me show you how.

About This Book

In this book I will try to explain my understanding of autism to other neurotypical people. Although I'll point out the kinds of differences you may find between us, I hope you will see that I am not saying one is better than the other. It is not better to be neurotypical, nor is it better to be Autistic.

It is best to be yourself.

I apologize in advance if this perspective is not always clear. There is a gulf between Autistic and neurotypical experiences, and in order to build a bridge of understanding, we need to look at that gulf head-on and consider many possibilities and points of view. I have to address the "inconvenient" aspects of autism, and at the same time consider just who it is inconvenient for: the Autistic person or the neurotypical people in their life. In other words, who is asking who to change, and why? Views on these issues vary all over the map and create unnecessary divides. I don't want to turn anyone into someone they are not, but I do want to make life easier for all. The gulf is wider than many people suspect, but I know from experience that a common understanding can be found.

Ironically, part of the gulf is a misunderstanding of how *alike* we really are. Most people assume there is something unusual about an Autistic child's emotional makeup. I am very concerned with the emotional world of Autistic children, but that's not where I see a big difference. Consider this: how would *you* react emotionally if you lived in a world you did not understand, where nobody understood you? Would you feel safe? What would you do to protect yourself? What I am suggesting is that many so-called "autistic behaviors" can be viewed as a normal reaction to life as a child experiences it. The child is reacting to a world most people do not see.

Goodness, you may think. *If that is true, then my child must have a really different view of day-to-day living.* Oh my, yes. To a child on the autism spectrum, the world does not look the same as it does to you or me. In some cases the differences are extreme. In part, this book is a tour of those differences. More than that, it is about how to discover them on your own. Take heart. When you get closer to the true way in which your child perceives things, then you can offer much more help than those who focus on the superficial. You will have in your hands the building blocks to bridge a gulf that many people barely accept or comprehend.

Again, with all this talk of a gulf between us, I don't want you to lose focus on our common human experience. I want you to feel compassion for the children who are trying to cross that gulf on their own in a society that does not fully recognize the true nature of their struggle. Underneath the neurological differences we are all still people. I hope this is as obvious to you as it is to me. You and your child can find ways to connect.

Who This Book Is About

This book is about the Autistic child (or children) in your life. Although the techniques are geared primarily toward children who are verbal or have emerging language, the philosophy behind the techniques applies across the spectrum. (This certainly includes children who have been diagnosed with Asperger's, even though, controversially, the diagnosis has been removed from the DSM-5.) There is something important here for anyone who knows an Autistic child.

At the risk of stating the obvious, I feel the need to emphasize that not all people on the autism spectrum are the same. When I give an example, please do not take it to apply to every Autistic child in the universe. It is not my intention to paint everyone with the same brush. I will try to point this out often, but I can't preface every statement with a disclaimer – you wouldn't want to read a book that was written like that! You will notice I often use words like *might*, *may*, and *can* as a reminder that no single example applies to everyone.

Speaking of the examples, privacy is of utmost importance in the field of mental health counseling, and I take it very seriously. As you can imagine, this presents a challenge when writing a book based on my experiences as a counselor. How can I provide you with useful real-life examples while protecting the privacy of those involved? Naturally the children's names have been changed. I have also altered identifying details while carefully preserving the essential truth of their stories. Some young adults actively want me to tell their stories; even in these cases certain details have been obscured out of consideration for how they might feel about it when they are five or ten years older. I will leave it to them to tell their own stories in their own way when the time is right. In the meantime, I've tried to imbue this book with the essence of their message as I have come to understand it.

This book is also about neurotypical people and how hard it is for us to understand autism. Obviously not all neurotypical people are the same, either. This book is about all of us – neurotypical and Autistic – and how we can all learn from each other.

Take what is helpful and build on it. There are ways to adapt for age, social understanding, and communication ability. The website given on the title page will be updated periodically with a broader range of examples. In the meantime, if you catch the philosophy behind the techniques, you should be able to adapt them to your child. Use age-appropriate tone. Use words your child understands. Do *not* assume your child has the social understanding expected for their age; a highly intelligent teenager may nonetheless need help with social understanding that is intuitive to most preschoolers. On the other hand, a child or teen with quite limited language can turn out to have a far richer intelligence than anyone has ever guessed. So do not assume anything is correlated in the way you'd expect.

By the way, I will not always say "child or teen." That is too cumbersome, so I will just say "child" even when the age range includes older children. I use the word to mean a person of any age up to adulthood. I hope this does not bother you if you're a teenager.

Who This Book Is For

This book is for anyone with an interest in autism, especially those who want to help a child on the autism spectrum be happy and connect with others. Clearly parents have a vested interest in their child's journey to social independence. So parents, I primarily address my words to you. I encourage everyone else in your child's life to read along and participate in the process. Aunts and uncles, teachers, counselors, aides, professionals of all kinds – this book is for you, too. It offers ideas about how we can all be more sensitive, more aware, and more helpful to children on the autism spectrum.

I hope you are patient with me. I have tried hard to choose my words carefully, but it has not always been easy. I do have a definite point of view. I want Autistic children to be happy. I am not trying to make them un-Autistic, nor am I trying to limit anyone in any way. If you want to better understand an Autistic child and improve the quality of their life, then I believe this book has something to offer.

Introduction

Safe and Understood

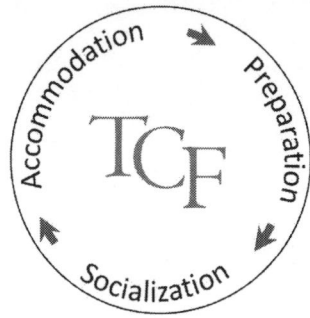

Interacting with the environment and the people in it involves social awareness that most of us take for granted. Imagine not being able to fit into the world around you no matter how hard you try.

1

Worlds Apart

When I was growing up there was a boy in the neighborhood who we all knew was "different." I'll call him Mark. Today I would say that Mark lacked the basic building blocks of social interaction, and might be diagnosed with ASD (Autism Spectrum Disorder). At the time I was only eight years old, trying to understand him and the way he was treated by others. I tried to put myself in his shoes.

Mark was teased mercilessly, depending on who was around. I wouldn't put up with it. My radar was on whenever he was nearby. I felt oddly responsible for him, though I was just another kid. Mainly, I remember wondering what life must be like for him.

Mark didn't know how to make or keep friends. Instead, he became a target. The neighborhood kids – even some of the nicest ones – would see how much they could get away with. For example, since Mark would believe anything you told him, kids would promise to play with him, and then ride off on their bikes, leaving him alone and waiting. The next day, he would believe the same story and wait some more. Mark always took things at face value, even when there was evidence to the contrary. He didn't understand the difference between friendly teasing and malicious mistreatment. He was an easy victim.

I began to ask, *Why?* Why is that happening? Why didn't others see that he couldn't help the way he was? Why couldn't he report the teasing to his parents? I came to understand that he didn't know how to accurately explain himself or describe a situation. The most obvious lie was seemingly too subtle for him. Perhaps it never occurred to him that people do not always tell the truth. Whatever the reason, he was easily outmaneuvered by his victimizers.

And I began to wonder why adults did not do more. How could it be okay to let life take him on this course while everyone just watches?

To this day, I still encounter adults who stand by and do nothing – and sometimes worse than nothing – because they don't understand what's going on. How far have we really come? Sometimes I wonder.

But the fact is that someone like Mark is not so easy to understand. I don't claim to have an instant way to understand every Autistic child through and through, but I have a pretty good working model and have found effective ways to adapt quickly. The key for me is this: *knowing that I don't know.* In many ways I am still like that eight-year-old, trying to figure things out. It may sound strange to say it this way, but I wish everyone would be a little less sure of themselves when it comes to autism. Paradoxically, this is a very confident stance. It can be uncomfortable to sit with uncertainty, but this is a far better starting point than being self-assured...and completely wrong. Knowing that you don't know brings its own kind of certainty. I always delve into new situations with absolute assurance that I do not know the whole story. That's how I get results. It's the challenge of the unknown that keeps me going. I have Mark to thank for this. I was both touched by compassion and intrigued by the mystery of his ways.

Indeed, Mark's behavior was truly mystifying to everybody. For example, when it was time for him to go home for supper, he would sometimes hide under our dining room table. Other days he would show up to play at sunrise, still in his pajamas. This is when the thought first occurred to me: If his behavior seems so strange to us, could our behavior seem just as strange to him? Does he wonder why he is welcome here at certain hours of the day, and at other times – well, not so much? Does he recognize the social cues of being welcome versus unwelcome, or even know that concept? Could he be unaware of the correlation between time of day and normal daily schedules? Did he know the difference between my home and his own? I began to consider the possibility that our behavior, so rational to us, might appear completely random to him. If he was missing even a few of these basic concepts then he would have no way to understand our world – not without our help.

In Mark's case I never found the answers. Yet I have come to rely on something even more important: finding the right questions. The answers differ from child to child; asking the right questions is key.

Of course as a kid I did not use words such as "social cues" and "missing concepts." What I do recall is that my thoughts took form as a mental image. I imagined two worlds, spinning in different directions, unable to make contact. We couldn't make sense of Mark's world, and he couldn't make sense of ours. That image stuck with me, and is an essential part of the work I do today.

My Perspective

I am a Licensed Mental Health Counselor who has worked with children and adults on the autism spectrum for over 25 years. In 2004 I founded The Friendship Network for Children, a nonprofit organization that applies The Connection Formula to improve the well-being of Autistic children and help them gain social independence. This is not your typical treatment facility for autism, in part because it is based on a component that others tend to omit: an absolute orientation toward understanding the child's point of view. A child-oriented view is the basis for this book, and it stems from a mental health perspective, so let me take a moment to explain.

A Licensed Mental Health Counselor (LMHC) is qualified to provide psychotherapy and diagnose depression, anxiety disorders, and other mental health concerns. In short, we are trained to deal with emotions. This is important because all sorts of emotional issues are usually right there in the mix with a child's autism.

Please don't misunderstand. I'm not saying that Autistic people have mental health issues as part of the diagnosis. What I am referring to is the human part of all of us – the part that has feelings, the part that makes connections with others, the part that can be impacted by extreme challenges and circumstances. So when I speak of the mental health perspective regarding a person on the autism spectrum, I am simply saying that their humanity is fully present. Obviously! One's humanity is completely intact for someone on the autism spectrum.

I also emphasize awareness of emotions because of the persistent myth that Autistic people lack feelings. Not only is this myth still alive and kicking, but it translates into how an Autistic person is treated by others. It's a recipe for insensitivity that goes something like this: If someone with autism has no feelings, then how can their feelings get hurt? Yikes! This misguided viewpoint leads down a very bad road.

> **The Emotional Mix**
>
> Dealing with emotions is a challenge for everyone. For some Autistic children, there are additional complications. Emotions are one more part of life that many children on the spectrum do not manage in a neurotypical way.
>
> Quite a few children have told me they do not understand why other therapists ask so many questions about feelings; these children do not see the role emotions play in the human experience. This is especially true of negative feelings – what I call the "unpopular" emotions. Many Autistic children are simply terrified of them.
>
> It is almost impossible to function in life without bringing emotions into the mix. We need to learn how to help without further frightening children on the autism spectrum with regard to emotions.

So to be perfectly clear, as a mental health professional I am saying that an Autistic person is a human being complete with feelings, and of course those feelings can be hurt. I see it happen almost every day, caused by people with the best of intentions. I am saying unequivocally that Autistic people have a wide range of feelings just like any human. This is so obvious to me that it took me a long time to figure out how to write this book. I didn't think it needed to be explained, but unfortunately it does.

Four Core Principles

The Connection Formula is more than a collection of techniques for parents. It's a therapeutic approach that mental health professionals can embrace, and it's a philosophy to guide that approach. This book presents aspects of my approach that parents can apply, explained in everyday language.

The techniques are important, but they mean little without the principles behind them. The core principles below may seem self-evident, but somehow they go missing when it comes to certain popular treatments for children on the autism spectrum. My purpose is to bring these principles front and center in everything we do. It is not necessary to be a therapist to apply them. They are for everyone. In whatever capacity you serve an Autistic child, The Connection Formula philosophy can enhance your work.

Core Principe #1:
Autistic children have feelings and want to connect with others

Autistic children feel happiness and sadness. They can feel hurt, they can feel betrayed. They can surely feel confused. They can feel a sense of loss. And Autistic children most definitely feel loneliness.

All of these emotions are in there. As a human, you have probably noticed that emotions can be rather complicated. Now, with autism, add to the mix any or all of the following:

➢ Difficulty self-soothing and regulating emotions

➢ A different way of understanding and using language

➢ Difficulty perceiving social norms

➢ Misconceptions about the purpose and nature of rules

➢ Sensory integration issues (sensitivity to sound, for example)

➢ Different ideas of cause and effect

➢ Unusual perceptions of time

Do these differences make it difficult to connect? They surely do. Some differences are so large that much of the world we take for granted might be entirely missing from the child's experience. That does not mean the child doesn't want to connect. Perhaps it is convenient to believe there are children who truly prefer to be isolated because it's just too heartbreaking to think otherwise.

An Autistic child may have tried to connect a thousand times – and may be trying still – only to have each attempt rejected because it is completely misunderstood. One young boy, hoping to connect with some older kids playing baseball in the street, took the stone they were using for home plate and dropped it down a nearby storm drain. Yes, he literally stole home base. As a result of actions like this, he was seen as the "weird kid," an outcast in the neighborhood. Nobody guessed he was simply trying to participate in the game and connect with others, so nobody showed him how.

The good news is that more people each day realize that Autistic children actually long to connect with others, even when outer appearances indicate otherwise. I would take this one step further: children on the spectrum *need* to connect. I may not be certain about much in this world, but I know that everyone needs to give and receive love. Autistic children choose isolation only because, without our help, they have no other option. No child is isolated by choice; the "choice" has been forced on them. The idea that these children want isolation is an old myth. We know better.

I've had the privilege to help many isolated children connect with others. In each case I look to see what took so long. What held them back? Perhaps a child had a bad experience in their first play date, say at age five. That child comes to me at age ten having never made a friend. Early failures can leave emotional wounds that linger indefinitely. Such wounds are in danger of being reopened on a daily basis. How does a child protect themselves? Some parents say, "Oh, they're happier playing video games." Other parents have tried time and again to hold successful play dates, and it just hasn't worked. In reality, these children are isolated by a gulf that they can't bridge on their own.

From a neurotypical point of view, we face this gulf whenever a child's actions don't make sense to us. Some confront the behavior directly; others give up in frustration. Still others look for the reasons behind the behavior, and that's the path we want to take.

Core Principle #2:
The world of an Autistic child has its own internal logic

When a child's actions don't seem to make sense to us, we should look for the underlying logic. Start by assuming that there *is* some underlying logic. We want to learn how your child experiences a moment.

I'm not saying that an Autistic child's logic is nonsensical. In fact, I am deeply humbled by just how logical some children are. The difficulty is often that their logic is based on a different premise from ours. When we try to interact, we use mismatched priorities. A whole new set of social weights and measures is in effect, which would be a manageable problem, except neither party seems to know that's what the problem is. As a result, Autistic children do not feel heard. They feel discounted. The neurotypical world underestimates the value of their point of view without really taking the time to understand it.

A child's internal logic will only start to make sense when you stop thinking "neurotypically" and recognize that there are these gaps – I call them *concept gaps* – between a generally accepted neurotypical viewpoint and the unique viewpoint of each Autistic child. You might be tempted to think of a concept gap as a child's misunderstanding of some social convention, and indeed that's often how a gap is spotted, but it really does go a lot deeper. If the premise behind a social convention is not intuitive to a child, then it won't make any sense to them. Where we see a logical pattern, a child on the spectrum might see only chaos. When they don't know the pattern, it's hard for them to fit in. As more than one Autistic person has expressed to me: *there are too many situations in life to memorize.* So the child is left to fill in patterns of their own. Then, if we miss their logic, we get to deal with our own fair share of chaos. We see it in the child's behavior. We see it in their way of interacting. We see it in the disrupted rhythms of daily life. Does this sound familiar?

People are too quick to dismiss a child's behavior as peculiar or nonsensical due to autism. Let's admit that this instinct can be wrong. Better to ask: *from what viewpoint does this behavior make sense*? That will lead you to the child's internal logic.

So please remember that confusion runs both ways. If you're confused by a child, how could they not be confused by you? Our world must make very little sense to some Autistic children. In fact, it might appear quite crazy. In their eyes, we are the peculiar ones. For some people this may be a new mindset. For me, investigating the internal logic of autism has become a way of life. I can tell you it is quite rewarding. Everyone wants to fix the chaos; first, let's understand the patterns behind it.

Core Principle #3:
Every child needs to feel safe and understood

Your child needs to feel safe and understood. Of course! You know this. But are the people who work with your child truly aware of all the implications? I'd be justified in calling this a "lost principle" because it has gone missing from so many interventions that treat the symptoms of autism without truly looking for the child within. For us it will be the starting point, and we never want to lose sight of it.

This principle is the gold standard by which you should evaluate any and all recommendations, including those in this book. If you can't apply a technique without causing your child distress, then don't do it. Your successes – and the happiness of your child – will be determined by how sacred you hold their emotional security.

Now you have the words to ask: *how will this help my child feel safe and understood?*

Core Principle #4:
Every child is worthy of love

This should hardly need an explanation, yet many treat Autistic children as broken, something to be fixed. What does that have to do with being worthy of love? Well, everything. When a child does not feel loved as they are, what message does it send?

We have to consider how things look from the child's point of view. Does society inculcate a "less-than" mentality about Autistic children? Some interventions can diminish a child's view of themselves. I have worked with a great many children whose self-esteem was negatively impacted. We do no service when we try to "fix" someone without understanding them. How do you imagine this feels to a child? Please, don't be a self-esteem stealer.

The approach I offer, the approach that helps a child feel safe and understood... and loved...can be summed up in three words: *connect before correct*. As a practical matter, this means you should understand your child before working on their behaviors.

Socialization is about forming authentic connections with others. If a child has difficulty connecting, we need to do the initial work to show them it is possible – *without behavioral preconditions*. We can create authentic connections with Autistic children just the way they are.

It is surely love that drives parents to try all they can to help their child. My question is: does the child know this? Unless love and acceptance are ingrained in the methodology itself, the answer may be *no*. Recognize the emotional impact of interventions that are geared toward correcting and changing a child. I'm not saying you shouldn't try to help your child. The right kind of help will build self-esteem and bring out positive changes from within.

I'm saying *lead with love*.

* * *

None of this will eliminate the need to consult with mental health professionals about your child. There is some fine print in the front of the book that talks about this. It has a message for anyone tempted to neglect a serious concern because they found a technique in a book – *any* book. The information I offer is to help you understand your child better; it is to enhance (not eliminate) all other avenues a reasonable person would pursue to get a child the help they need. I hope this book leads you to better understand the help that's needed, but even here we tread into territory best left to experts when serious concerns are afoot. In particular, you will sense my LMHC initials coming to the fore whenever I'm on the topic of anxiety and depression, which need to be assessed and treated by a qualified professional.

The Connection Formula is not just to help you understand autism; it's to help your child understand *you* as you adapt your parenting style to their needs. It's a style that is not widely known, in part because the psychotherapy model has not had a big role in shaping popular techniques. Traditional practitioners who work with Autistic children seem unfamiliar with one or more principles that I consider absolutely essential, and this ties right in with my concerns about anxiety and depression. To be blunt: many common practices can do more harm than good. I want you to know why. When you internalize the four core principles above, you'll be a more effective watchdog for your child's well-being.

I like the Autistic people in my life and enjoy spending time with them, just as I do with neurotypical people. I feel compassion, love, and support from them. It never occurred to me to think they do not have feelings or that they are somehow broken. Sadly, there are too many people who still hold a different view.

The Connection Formula does not attempt to make somebody into something they are not. Quite the contrary, when children feel safe and understood – when they feel love and acceptance – a great weight is lifted and they are free to become more themselves.

2

The Compassion Gap

Imagine that you overhear the following exchange between a parent and child outside a restaurant.

Parent:	Justin, get up these stairs so we can all go inside and eat.
Justin:	I can't.
Parent:	Can't or won't?
Justin:	Can't.
Parent:	Don't be ridiculous. I'll let you have extra dessert if you get up here right now.
Justin:	(Starts to cry.)
Parent:	THAT'S ENOUGH! No dinner for you tonight – and no video games for a week.

On the surface it seems obvious what's going on here. A family's evening out has been disrupted. A parent tries some typical techniques to coax their child up the stairs and into the restaurant, but nothing seems to work. Overhearing this exchange, we get the impression of an uncooperative child in need of some behavioral intervention. Well turn around and look at the whole picture. Justin is in a wheelchair, and there is no access ramp in sight.

Surprised? It would be very disturbing to witness a scene like this in real life. You would wonder, *where is the compassion*? Fortunately this is a made-up story to illustrate a point. Unfortunately, the point is this: such a scene plays out all the time, except the child's obstacle is invisible. We cannot blame the parents for missing it, because how are they to know?

Many professionals also miss the obstacles that Autistic children face. This unfortunate reality is driven home by experiences like the following. I was at a school giving a talk to parents and educational professionals. A great deal of my presentation was about using accommodations to create a foundation of mutual understanding between the adults and the students on the spectrum – essentially the first part of The Connection Formula (although I did not have this name for it at the time). I was sharing some stories to help make my point – illustrating how very different the world looks through the eyes of an Autistic child and how far we must go to help them feel safe and understood – when the director of special education rather curtly interrupted and said, "We understand what these kids are all about. We don't need any more descriptions of them."

Well I had worked with some students from that school, and knew firsthand how misunderstood those children were. They did not feel safe there, and had suffered emotional consequences that became my job to treat. Yet somehow the emotional well-being of the children – and the consequences of ignoring their stress level – were completely invisible to some individuals in the room. They were looking right at the problem, and just couldn't see it. As a result, the well-meaning staff appeared cruel and abusive to the children.

That is the compassion gap.

The sad irony is that the school was undermining their own purpose by using an approach that negated everything they hoped to accomplish. When children are emotionally wounded because we do not make the effort to understand them, we have a very serious problem.

Autistic children stand at the foot of an insurmountable obstacle while adults try to coax them to the top, somehow putting the burden on the child to reach the goals that we have set. Of course this is all done with the best of intentions. The gulf of understanding is so great that few can believe traditional approaches are so far off the mark. Frustration grows, and the gulf gets wider. When you glimpse the truth of what is really going on, the compassion gap is obvious and shocking.

To bridge the gap, you need to understand the nature of the

obstacles these children face. Obviously Justin will not have access to that restaurant without our help. What is it that Autistic children need help accessing? It is social information.

What Is Social Information?

Social information is information about our neurotypical reality. All of it.

Think of everything you know about how the world works, from the smallest social interaction (like chatting with a stranger at a bus stop) to the largest institutions (governments, hospitals, school systems), and everything in between. Social information ranges from the most basic concepts (you are you and I am me) to the most complex social interactions (applying to college, finding a job, buying a home, dealing with all sorts of organizations and officials). And of course, it includes meeting people and connecting with them.

All of us are missing information in one area or another, but we manage to get by using the ability to learn general principles about one scenario and carry that knowledge forward, adapting it to another. For example, not everyone is good at making travel reservations or getting a good deal when buying a car. Still, we will recognize that these are established systems that work by their own rules – even if we don't know what the rules are. On the other hand, most of us know some basics, like the ordering procedure in a typical restaurant or how to wait in line at a movie theater. And although we can be temporarily thrown when encountering a new system, we will usually cope with the unfamiliar and adjust. Often we adapt by knowing when and how to ask for help – another social interaction.

All of this – the structure of the world and how we think of it – comprises our neurotypical reality. You would be hard-pressed to explain it in full to anyone because it's too big, you don't know all of it, and much of what you do know is so ingrained that you seldom think about it.

Fortunately you don't have to explain all of it. However, depending on your child, you may be called on to explain the hardest parts. Can you guess what those are? The hardest things to explain are the "you are you and I am me" kind of fundamentals. This can be difficult because these are probably not things you ever thought you'd need to discuss. A child on the spectrum might be able to describe why the sky is blue, and you would come away knowing a little something about the light-scattering characteristics of earth's atmosphere. On the other hand, you might find it difficult to explain why it's okay – indeed, how it's even possible – for two people to have different favorite colors. Chances are that nobody needed to explain it to *you*, so it can be hard to come up with the right words. And for most neurotypical people it's harder still to recognize and accept that something so basic might need to be explained at all.

I use the term *social information* mainly to refer to information at that basic level, but it is broad enough to cover the whole continuum of neurotypical reality and all the rules, procedures, and conventions in it. The social information that you will need to explain to an Autistic child can include any and all details about how the world works, but most frequently you'll find that it has to do with the interactions we have with each other. It's even important to include interactions with inanimate objects. A child's difficulty with a car door, a button, a zipper – even a game or toy – may deeply affect how they think about themselves and their place in the world.

Because the kind of social information you need to convey tends toward those difficult basics – the things we take for granted – it is harder to find common ground. It's easier for people to relate on topics that confuse *everyone*. It's much harder when you assume someone knows something they don't. It's like speaking two different languages without realizing it.

For neurotypical children we have a system in place for understanding how a child perceives social information; therefore, we know how to teach and reinforce social learning, or at least we move generally in the right direction. If a neurotypical child can't share a toy or argues with a friend, there are a variety of interventions and strategies adults use, often without consciously thinking about it. You might see a mom at a playground encouraging young children to take turns. You'll hear a dad say, "You are such a nice big brother." Parents will step in to quell an argument between two sisters at a restaurant. You get the idea; the list of neurotypical strategies is long. Of course it doesn't always work perfectly, but we have a well-travelled road when the child's reality matches our neurotypical assumptions. The neurotypical child can conceptually and emotionally receive social information and then independently bring it forward. In other words, the child can generalize and learn socially from daily interactions. No one really even stops to think about a neurotypical child's social learning ability at this very basic level. It's a given and is taken for granted.

A child on the autism spectrum has a different social learning style. They do not learn and bring the social information forward independently the way neurotypical children do. You can think of this as a *social learning disability*.

> **What Is a Social Learning Disability?**
>
> The term refers to connection and communication issues, and is often applied to children on the autism spectrum. It's a way to describe people who don't pick up on social cues at the level of their peers. Although not currently an official diagnosis, the term does convey a sense of the challenges faced by Autistic children who are disconnected from our everyday social reality. Perhaps *disability* is the right word. Perhaps not. People in the field seem to be struggling to find the best terminology (to wit, the disappearance of the Asperger's diagnosis from the DSM-5), so let's not get too hung up on the terms in vogue at the time of this writing.
>
> I'll use the term *social learning disability* even though it may fall out of favor by the time you read this. It's more important to develop your own instinctive sense of what it's like in the Autistic world...to the extent that we can even say there is an "Autistic world," for in truth each child's world is different. You won't get to the heart of your child's experience by memorizing a definition; you need to catch the deeper sense of reality behind the descriptive words we use.

There is a dearth of information about the social-emotional development of children on the autism spectrum. Nobody is quite sure what's going on. As a broad generalization let's say that their processing of social information works differently from what people expect. I don't make a judgment about whether it is better or worse. It's just different. The consequences for being so different in a world that does not understand can be extreme. Even a "mild" social learning disability can create an environment in which you are severely misunderstood. Many simply suffer in silence, cut off from life through no choice of their own.

For an Autistic child, that is a big stairway to climb.

Our neurotypical social ways need to be addressed in a manner that makes sense to someone with a social learning disability, in a way that allows them to feel safe and understood.

To take it a step further, social information isn't just about two people interacting; it's about interactions with the world in general. Systems such as government, community, customs, and laws also need to be addressed in a manner that makes sense to the Autistic child. When our neurotypical logic meets an unknown in the neurotypical world, we go through a neurotypical process of adapting. Mainly, we match new situations with things we have already learned. We spot the gaps in our own knowledge and figure out how to fill those gaps. We do some research. We ask for help.

Now what can we say about an Autistic child in this scenario? First, their perception of the world may be different, so what exactly are they adapting to – the world as it is or the world as they see it? Second, their internal logic may be different. What conclusions will they reach? What options will they consider? A child might not see how past experiences can be generalized to fit the new situation. They might not know the concept of asking for help, or may lack the ability to accurately report their problem. Third, we have to consider the emotional impact on the child as they try to cope. You are dealing with a rich, multi-layered reality that can be surprisingly unlike the familiar world you know.

For a child it is just plain scary.

* * *

So when I talk about conveying social information, I am talking about all of the above: the vast amount of information – including basic concepts – which you cannot take for granted; the layers of "ASD reality" that the information must be adapted to; and the child's emotional readiness to deal with each and every facet of life as they encounter it.

Now I am absolutely not saying that every Autistic child is missing every piece of social information. Of course not! I am simply saying that most people do not stop to consider the scope of social information that might be missing. Before we can bring two worlds together, we have to recognize how far apart they actually are.

Get to Know Your Child's World

We need to make life accessible to Autistic children because it's not reasonable to make them do it on their own. You need an access ramp to join your worlds. In practical terms, this means you will need to make some adjustments in your language, activities, and routines so that you and your child can understand each other.

But to build an access ramp for socialization, you first need to meet the child where they are – at ground level, so to speak. If you start the ramp at step three and your child is stuck at step one, it doesn't do them much good, does it? That is why I say *get to know your child's world*. What is this invisible obstacle that is so hard for your child to overcome? We should always be looking for it. There may be a gap of understanding far bigger than you think. I know this from countless interactions with Autistic children, yet I am always surprised when I uncover a new concept gap.

> ➤ Alicia is a bright student on the autism spectrum. Her parents encourage her to study in order to do well in school, but her study habits lead to mixed results. She may study science the night before a history test, or memorize the spelling of the big cats of the savannah to prepare for a math quiz. Teacher and parents are looking for neurotypical problems of motivation and attention, but Alicia simply does not perceive cause and effect the way we do. She literally does not recognize how study of a subject relates to performance in a test on that subject, and she reacts strongly against accepting any help in this area. It seems that our neurotypical approach makes no sense to her. For Alicia,

study involves a unique sort of logic that leads to all sorts of misunderstandings. We clearly have a concept gap here, and work is needed to fully uncover it.

- Eric has a meltdown with nearly every transition, from leaving for school in the morning to going to bed at night. Like many of us, his parents struggle with time management, so they see his behavior as a version of their own difficulty meeting schedules. But Eric's difficulties are not just an exaggerated version of a neurotypical problem. Eric is deeply confused by time itself. He doesn't seem to understand that the passage of time is not under our control. When the sun comes up and it's time for school, he is not merely grumbling about an early schedule. At a deep level, beyond his own ability to articulate it, he might be reacting to the inexplicable cruelty of parents who do not hold back the sunrise. Is this literally how he thinks? I cannot say for sure. I do know that life gets extraordinarily confusing for all concerned when a child does not see the difference between what we can and cannot control.

- Pete is a teenager who stayed home alone one afternoon while his mother ran a quick errand. He needed a pencil for his school work, and found one in the family supply drawer. However, he was later filled with bad feelings for "stealing" the pencil. We had to deal with his anxiety at his next therapy session. You see, Pete has a great deal of difficulty understanding why different rules apply in different places. At school he would need permission to take a pencil. He has been reassured that the pencils at home are there for his use, but the concept still does not fit his internal logic. He has to memorize each exception to his intuitive grasp of life. Will all these exceptions eventually gel into a new logical pattern, or will Pete forever struggle in a world full of contradictions? Time will tell. This is Pete's journey, and he is making steady progress, overcoming one misunderstanding at a time.

The Compassion Gap

Recall the words of that special education director I mentioned at the beginning of this chapter. "We understand what these kids are all about." You do? Really? He and his staff had not begun to guess what children like Alicia, Eric, and Pete were all about. Yet to get started, that is all you really need to do. *Begin to guess.*

I make educated guesses all the time in order to get to the bottom of each situation. Perhaps I am more open than most to "out of the box" ideas about how a child might perceive the world. This gets me past my own neurotypical blinders, and more quickly leads to the truth of the matter, or at least something closer to the truth. Guessing wrong is not a problem as long as you are willing to immediately try another idea if your theory does not pan out. I am always telling children, "Oh, that is my mistake." And we go forward from there. I can assure you they appreciate the effort.

Now certainly the process I use involves a lot more than just guessing, but I will tell you that imagination is a big part of it. It is helpful to generate a steady stream of ideas so that when one does not work, you can quickly move on to another. And here at the outset, I hope to open your mind and heart to a full appreciation of the gulf that we are asking these children to cross – even if you have to guess about it as you get started.

We begin with the obvious goal: help a child socialize and be happy. However, we need to back up the process a few steps to find the child's ground level and provide an access ramp that they can reach. This is why we don't confront behavior in a traditional way. Focusing on behavior alone does not make life accessible. Instead, we try any accommodations we can think of to reach the child in their world, so that we can give them access to ours.

You don't need me to make you a compassionate person. I know you want to help. I want to help you show your compassion in a way your child can recognize and accept.

3

What Is the Connection Formula?

Socialization is not just about going to parties or playing with friends. Every interaction is a social interaction. Interacting with the environment and the people in it involves social awareness that most of us take for granted. Imagine not being able to fit into the world around you no matter how hard you try.

It's hard for an Autistic child to socialize because they lack some fundamental social information, and because it is difficult for us to determine – and accept – just how much help is needed. For example, you may wish to teach about taking turns in a game, but does the child understand what makes a game different from other activities? When was the last time *you* thought deeply about what makes a game a game? There is some sort of goal involving rules and structure, with a beginning, middle, and end. Sounds easy, but does the child know these concepts? Time and structure and rules may be unclear; some concepts could simply be absent. Which concepts will you need to teach? How will you find out?

Some children will have complete confidence in their understanding of a game, even when it is quite disconnected from the way everyone else plays. A child may in fact live by a set of fundamental rules known only to them. And like most people, they assume their basic concepts are the same for everyone. Now *you* are the one missing some fundamental social information about *their* world. Remember Alicia and her unusual study logic or Pete and his guilt over breaking a non-existent pencil rule. In addition to missing concepts, we have extra concepts. Hidden concepts.

These are all examples of concept gaps, where a child's internal logic does not match up with established norms. How far will you get if your approach to teaching social information doesn't match itself to a child's logic? My observation: not very far.

And there's another challenge: the ever-present emotional component. Think of a child who emotionally shuts down when they get confused. What if you want to teach about the importance of listening when someone talks? Can you assume the child has no confusion regarding the concept of communication? Do they even know why people have conversations? Some children literally do not see the point of it. They might not perceive a difference between questions and answers. They might construe the whole interaction in a novel way. Your attempts to teach a lesson can be a giant source of confusion to such a child, and then *you* become confused by the child's emotional reaction. This is surely not a recipe for success.

Consider possibilities like these and you will begin to understand how far we need to step back from our neurotypical assumptions.

Socialization 3-2-1

For all the reasons above, social information needs to be broken down and delivered in ways you may have never considered. Working backwards, it goes like this:

3

Most people want to start with the basics of socialization, but the "basics" are not basic enough. The child does not respond in the way we expect, and neurotypical teaching methods do not seem to help. The child is not conceptually or emotionally prepared to handle what we have to offer, so we have to back up a step.

2

To prepare the child, we need to learn what is going on from their perspective in order to correctly identify their areas of need. Now we find that communication is unreliable. We just don't know what the child needs because we are not speaking the same language.

So, one more step back.

What Is the Connection Formula?

1

We find ways to communicate by using literal language, visual aids like a problem scale, and many other accommodations that give us insights while helping the child to feel safe and understood. Now we are getting somewhere! Progress begins.

* * *

Putting things in proper order, we have the three parts of The Connection Formula: Accommodation, Preparation, and Socialization. Let me introduce you to them.

Part 1: Accommodation

We begin with accommodations. For someone with a hearing disability, we want to make communication accessible. For someone with disabled mobility, we want to make the environment accessible. For someone who is blind, we have many accommodations (from service dogs to sophisticated technologies) to make life accessible.

Well, more than accessible. Convenient. Enjoyable.

Perhaps the most apt and obvious symbol of accessibility is the wheelchair access ramp. We are not surprised to see them, and have come to expect this accommodation. When it comes to autism – a social learning disability – it is natural to think about how we can make socialization accessible. So where are the access ramps for those with a social learning disability? What accommodations are available for children with ASD? There are a great many. Here is a sampling from Part 1 of the book:

> ➢ **Language accommodations** (and common sense) tell us to adopt a literal communication style when working with someone who thinks in a literal way. For example:
>   o Be careful with idioms
>   o Avoid sarcasm
>   o Abbreviate language
>
> ➢ **Feeling accommodations** make emotions less scary and give your child safe ways to communicate about them. These accom-

modations are based on the idea of leading with facts before addressing feelings:

- Put comments before questions
- Give concrete choices
- Play the *true or false* game
- Use feeling phrases
- Find connecting logic

➢ **Visual accommodations** use pictures and graphics to enhance communication. A visual rating system can help a child clarify their viewpoint in many areas, using scales like these:

- The safety scale
- The logic scale
- Feeling scales
- The problem pyramid

These are especially useful in combination with other accommodations, and give a proactive way to reduce anxiety. We want a child to feel safe *before* they react to stress, and so we give them tools to show us how they think and feel.

➢ **Accommodations for sequencing** build on logic and facts as a way to comfort and connect. The idea is to put factual information in a logical sequence to make life predictable. Sequencing helps to:

- Explain plans and schedules
- Calm your child's fears
- Review a day's events
- Uncover your child's view of past, present, and future

Accommodations begin with you, but they are not one-sided. Children can learn to use them independently. Introduce them to your child to build reliable communication for both of you. When communication is reliable at home, you can look to the wider world and imagine new possibilities.

How do we bring things forward? At the risk of repeating myself: preparation, preparation, preparation.

Part 2: Preparation

Here we deal with two questions: Where will the accommodations lead you? And: how will you lead your child? The first question has to do with discovering your child's internal logic and the path it takes them on; the second relates to course corrections to help your child navigate daily life.

The theme here is *Connect Before Correct* because it reminds us to put accommodations first. Accommodations build connections on many levels:

- ➢ A connection to your child's way of perceiving and thinking about the world;

- ➢ A connection to the social input that your child needs;

- ➢ A connection to your child's emotional readiness for change;

- ➢ A connection to your child themselves, so they see you as someone who understands them and can help.

Connections allow us to be meaningful with the social information we convey, and protective in our manner of conveying it. Quite unknowingly, people fail to connect to a child's point of view, and then compound the problem by reacting insensitively to the disorientation they cause. The child feels betrayed, if I may use such a word to describe what many children have tried to explain to me. We betray their logic and we betray their emotions. Let's not do that anymore. Instead, be a guardian for your child's point of view, even as you move them toward understanding yours. Connect before correct.

A tall order? Yes, it certainly can be. We'll need more accommodations for teaching social information, but the Preparation stage has as much guidance for you as it does for your child. It shows how to:

- ➢ Recognize concept gaps

- ➢ Own misunderstandings

- ➢ Reprogram your responses

The Connection Formula

> ➢ Unconfuse the rules
>
> ➢ Be a proactive problem solver

When you succeed, your child will believe in something new and life-changing: the possibility of a trusted ally who understands them and keeps them safe. That's the backdrop you want to create for social learning. The goal is to move your child forward in a way that connects with their logic, their feelings, and their needs.

Part 3: Socialization

The third part of the formula involves building friendships and socialization skills. At this stage we can finally address what most people think of as the basics, like taking turns in a game or listening to a friend who is talking. This is where many people start, but as I have explained, skipping the earlier steps is asking too much of a child on the autism spectrum. With all your preparation in place, let's survey the work to do and the possibilities now in reach.

> ➢ **Become your child's social coach.** Think about the many roles you play as a parent, and blend this one into the mix. It's a way to stay calm and know your intention.
>
> ➢ **Create shared moments.** They connect us all, but you and your child will likely have very different frames of reference. What does it mean to prove the value of a moment to your child? Food for thought: your child may be trying to do the same with you.
>
> ➢ **Implement Family Fun Time**, a microcosm for socialization in the home. Flexible structure calms your child by accommodating their areas of need while making social expectations clear. It's a prerequisite for successful play dates.
>
> ➢ **Learn social choreography.** This means thinking in details about social interactions and their natural rhythm that might not come naturally at all to an Autistic child. Family Fun Time will give you lots of practice!

What Is the Connection Formula?

> **Social independence** is our goal. You'll need a yardstick to gauge the social freedom your child can responsibly handle. Important components include:
> - Valid reporting
> - Acceptance of feedback
> - Self-advocacy
> - Self-observation

> **A successful play date** is a big milestone. What does it take to plan one? Everything you and your child have learned comes into play. This is our final milestone in this book, but for many children it can be the start of authentic friendships and rewarding social interactions.

The three parts of The Connection Formula need to be revisited in a cyclical way. That's why they are represented in a circle. Each part builds on the others, bringing new insights and new ways to move forward.

(Diagram: a circle labeled TCF with Accommodation, Preparation, and Socialization arranged around it.)

Knowing Your Intention

Knowing your intention means being clear about your goals. It also means being clear about the attitude required to connect with your child. So when I speak about *intention*, I am referring to a particular perspective about autism that is important to keep foremost in your mind – not just while you read this book, but also when you interact with your child, when you think about your child, and when you talk with others about your child. Why is this necessary? It's because there is a strong tendency to slip back into neurotypical thought patterns. A conscious effort is required to autism-ize your thinking and maintain that point of view.

> When working with other clinicians, I will often say, "Let's back up." We have to stop and back up our thinking in 3-2-1 style to peel away assumptions. The "Aha!" moments come when we back up far enough to gain perspective on our own neurotypical blind spots.
>
> The way I look at it, we have accepted an important mission, and we hold the intention of fulfilling it. Aligning yourself with a clear sense of purpose allows you to apply what you are learning even when natural neurotypical responses pull you in the wrong direction.

The Essential First Step

Every child needs to feel safe and understood. This is common sense backed up by developmental psychology. Think about it. We all need to feel safe and understood. Of course! It sure feels a lot better than the alternative. It's a happy state of mind, it's emotionally healthy, and it's the best starting point for anything else you might want to accomplish.

Think about what it means for you to feel safe and understood. For example, consider the misunderstandings that can arise at work. Have you ever been misunderstood by a coworker? Perhaps the boss underestimated the complexity of a task, and reprimanded you for taking too long. Or maybe you were unfairly blamed for a mistake. How would you feel in such a situation? "Safe and understood" is probably not the first phrase to come to mind. Until the situation is resolved, it can feel like a struggle to survive in the workplace.

What about relationships with friends or family members? How do you get back to a comfortable equilibrium when your feelings have been hurt? If you feel safe in the relationship, you can talk things through and try to make your feelings known. Given the messiness of human emotions the result is never guaranteed, but if you're at least somewhat successful you will manage to express your feelings and hopefully come to a new balance with your loved ones.

I'm sure you can think of many such examples from your own life, though perhaps you haven't thought of them in terms of feeling safe and understood. A neurotypical person's ability to navigate these situations is so ingrained that we seldom consider all that is involved. Once again, I'm talking about fundamental neurological abilities – for example, the ability to understand language, to determine what people expect of us, even the ability to perceive others as separate individuals with their own point of view. All are abilities we assume to be present in everyone, but these are just a few of the many areas where autism can impact a child's way of being in the world, leaving them in a fight for emotional survival. Navigating tricky interactions can be difficult for all of us. For an Autistic child, every interaction is potentially tricky because the neurological makeup that we take for granted is just plain different. Even the ability to identify their own inner struggle and pinpoint its source is something children on the autism spectrum often lack.

I hear recommendations like this: *fix their behavior and they will be happy.* But behavior is only superficial evidence of the underlying problem. It sure would be convenient if you could flip a switch, modify a behavior, and make your child happy. Nothing is so cut and dried, but you *can* flip your viewpoint. Look for the true obstacles to your child's happiness. Just as all mobility accommodations have the goal of helping someone move from here to there, a common goal of our ASD accommodations is to help a child feel safe and understood so they can move toward social independence.

No approach works well if your child must climb a wall of anxiety and confusion in order to meet your expectations. On the other hand, if you can accommodate their need to feel safe and understood, little miracles are possible. Helping your child feel safe and understood is the essential first step of each and every interaction.

Aim for the Possible

You may know Lao-tzu's famous saying, "The journey of a thousand miles begins with a single step." This seems like small consolation when you feel you have so far to go, but there is another way to look at it: see and enjoy the value of each step. I found an alternate translation that comes closer to this spirit: "The journey of a thousand miles begins beneath one's feet."

You can enjoy your child with each step along the way.

The Connection Formula

* * *

While waiting in line to board a plane, I noticed an Autistic boy standing with his family just on the other side of a little half-height dividing wall made of transparent glass tiles. The boy seemed to be quite within his own world as he lifted his hand and pressed it flat against one of the tiles. On instinct, I pressed my own hand against my side of the same tile, mirroring the position of his hand against the glass. When the boy moved his hand to a different tile, I moved mine to match. We repeated this pattern a few times. Then I pressed my hand to a different tile, and on his side the boy followed in kind, exactly mirroring mine. Sometimes the boy led, sometimes I led. Always our hands mirrored each other against the transparent tiles. This game continued for perhaps a half a minute before the boarding process ended our interaction. We never said a word.

That is the whole Connection Formula philosophy in a thirty second encounter. Do you see a rhythm to it? I don't want to over-explain – we have the rest of the book ahead of us for you to catch the spirit of what I'm trying to put across. The techniques are quite concrete; the intention behind them is very subtle. For now let's just say that the progression of this encounter represents the three parts of the formula: entering the child's world, leading them to ours, and feeling the heart of a real connection. It has to do with shared moments, and that is what we are always trying to achieve. One shared moment followed by another, and another. Each shared moment brings things forward for us and the child. The long-term goals matter, but shared moments matter more.

It begins beneath your feet.

I will set no limits about what might be possible down the road for any child. As a practical matter, it's important to determine what is possible at this point in the journey. Each time you achieve some small goal, you set the stage for the next one. Aim for the possible. In this way you can enjoy continuous progress.

Part 1: Accommodation

Making Life Accessible

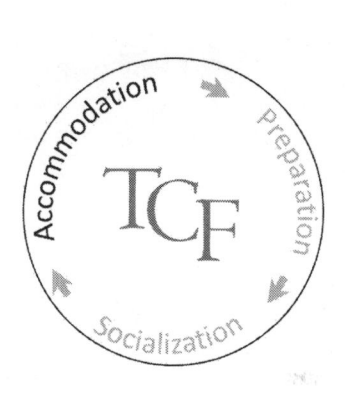

Accommodations get you close enough to your child for them to accept the tools you have to offer. Then you will be able to guide, nurture, and parent your child towards social independence.

4

Watch Your Language

It's easy to take language for granted because we learn it so naturally. A neurotypical child has fun by playing with language, making up silly words or rhymes. Even very young children can pick up common idioms. Of course at times unfamiliar expressions and vocabulary need to be explained to neurotypical children; that's part of the development process. In general, you will find that a neurotypical child understands language more or less at the same level as their peers.

This is not true for someone on the autism spectrum. Idioms and common expressions can be very confusing, so we make adjustments in our communication style, being watchful for pragmatic language issues such as difficulty understanding the meaning of words, grammar, and syntax. What is the nature of these difficulties? When trying to imagine what this must be like for Autistic children, neurotypical people tend to think of their own ability to learn new vocabularies (or a whole new language) and project an exaggerated version of the challenge onto the child. "Oh, it's hard for me to remember a new expression, maybe it's ten times harder for my child." It's an empathetic response, a good start toward closing the compassion gap. However, such comparisons can miss the true nature of the situation. It is not necessarily a matter of degree; sometimes it's a matter of kind. Here's what I mean: You probably think in language; if so, words are part of your thought process. However, what if a child thinks in pictures? Or concepts? Or intent? This is a completely different kind of challenge. Translation to and from words is surely a cumbersome process for someone whose thoughts are not framed in language.

But even that is not the whole story. There are two levels to the language difficulties that you might encounter: processing of language itself, and the reasoning that goes on beneath the surface (the child's internal logic). A common language is of limited value when you lack a common frame of reference for the reasoning behind it, but you won't be able to establish that frame of reference without working your way through the language difficulties. We have to work our way through one layer at a time, and so we'll begin with language accommodations, while always keeping the larger perspective in mind.

Be Careful with Idioms

For a child on the autism spectrum, a simple conversation can be a minefield. When your literal meaning diverges from your intended meaning, you create confusion. In some cases idioms can even be hurtful. If a word or phrase has a negative connotation for a child, it can overpower the intended meaning of the idiom. I know children who have had strong negative reactions to phrases like these:

- See you later, alligator
- I'd give my right arm
- I'll keep my eye on you
- I'm itching to go
- I have a frog in my throat
- You hit the nail on the head
- We have to kill some time
- A tongue in cheek remark
- Don't be a stranger
- Don't let the bedbugs bite
- Don't let the cat out of the bag

We take idioms like these in stride, but stop and consider the literal words and the images they conjure: hitting and killing; losing an arm; a disembodied eye; a dislocated tongue; biting bugs and invasive frogs; strangers and alligators and that poor cat. Even if a child understands a figure of speech, their internal logic might still see and process the literal imagery. Imagine trying to process two contradictory meanings at the same time; then add in the difficulty of overcoming the emotional reaction to a strange or unpleasant image. Many children have asked me, "Why can't people just say what they mean?"

Here is how I have answered:

> *Sometimes people use expressions that don't make sense to explain their thoughts. It can be very confusing! I'm not always sure why people do this. There is usually a historical reason for the expression, but not everyone understands it. The person is not trying to be confusing. People are not always 100% logical in how they talk or how they think.*

Even on hearing a figure of speech for the first time, you can usually catch its meaning based on the context. What if you lacked this ability? Imagine that the context itself eluded you, or simply evaporated in confusion. In an instant an Autistic child can lose their grip on the social interaction (if they had such a grip in the first place) and zoom in on something that other people might not even notice. One detail gets all the attention, out of proportion to the actual situation. This can happen with anything – colors, objects, sounds, smells – and it certainly happens with idioms. A word with a negative connotation can trump reality, causing a child to lose trust in the world.

How a child handles these misunderstandings will vary widely. That is the nature of the minefield of language – you just don't know what will trigger a negative reaction. *Overreaction*, some might say. But remember, *you are simply not perceiving the world in the same way as the child*. A child might feel safe in the moment, then a word or phrase disrupts their tenuous connection to safety. Panic is a perfectly understandable reaction when one's reality is turned upside-down. Not all reactions will be so extreme, thank goodness.

Hopefully you're starting to see some ways in which language difficulties feed into the underlying logic of autism. Even a simple phrase like "take a seat," when interpreted literally, can lead to embarrassment. How would you feel if you risked such a misunderstanding in practically every interaction of your life? It's not hard to understand why a child would withdraw from social interactions.

So be careful with idioms. Many children on the spectrum can become extraordinarily frustrated with them, and have difficulty tolerating them emotionally.

How can you help? Simplify language. Explain idioms when you use them, and avoid them in stressful situations. Some children have developed a good sense of idioms, but when in new situations, the meanings evade them. It's wise to completely avoid idioms when talking to an Autistic child who is under stress.

Here is how I explain some common idioms:

> **Time flies**
>
> *Time flies, but not like the clock will get wings on it and fly across the room. Many things that fly – like birds and airplanes – can move really fast. People say 'time flies' when it seems like time is moving really fast.*

> **That stinks!**
>
> *This does not mean something smells bad and you need to hold your nose. Well, sometimes that is exactly what it means if your nose smells something you don't like. Other times when people say 'That stinks!' they are using these words to explain an experience that is uncomfortable or awkward, or to say that a situation is unpleasant – just like a bad smell. Even though it doesn't smell bad to your nose, it is still unpleasant.*

> **See you later alligator**
>
> *I know you are not an alligator, that you are a person. People like to say this expression because 'alligator' rhymes with 'later' and they think it sounds good. The sound became popular. That means many people liked hearing and saying the rhyme. The*

> rhyme makes people happy so they repeat the expression even though humans are not alligators.
>
> It is another way of saying goodbye. And sometimes they don't even plan to see you later. Now that really doesn't make sense!

Here's an expression that you might need to explain to a teenager or older child:

> **You'll always be in my heart**
>
> This does not mean I think you will become a miniature being living in the heart that is in my body. That would be very inconvenient for both of us! (That's a joke, because it's not even possible.)
>
> 'In my heart' means I have feelings that are very strong in a good, positive way. Sometimes it means the feeling of love. So, I will remember you in a positive way with a powerful feeling of goodness. I will not think about you all the time. I will think of you intermittently for the rest of my life. When I do think about you it will always be in this positive way.

See if you can come up with explanations for figures of speech that you frequently use. If you can't think of any off the top of your head, here are a few to try. (And "off the top of your head" is another one.)

- Cut it out
- Hold your horses
- When pigs fly
- Don't be fresh
- It's a piece of cake
- See eye to eye

It's not always so easy to do! All the more reason to be careful with idioms. If you can't explain one, it is best to avoid it.

The Connection Formula

You might be surprised how often you use idioms without being aware of it. Learning to spot them can be a fun family game. Turn on the TV and start counting, or observe two family members having a conversation. This can be quite enjoyable as you try to picture what some phrases would look like if they really happened, like "it's raining cats and dogs."

> **Bring in the Laughter**
>
> Bring in the laughter, but be careful not to laugh *at* someone when an idiom is misunderstood, because that can be extremely humiliating.
>
> In general, be careful with humor. When using humor, state you are doing so. For example, say, "I am being silly right now." Or simply state, "That was a joke."

For elementary school children, I recommend the *Amelia Bedelia* series of books by Peggy Parish. The main character continuously misunderstands figures of speech, with comical results. It's a lighthearted way to introduce the topic of idioms and the confusion they cause. These books can be fun for the whole family.

Provide a safe and fun environment to allow your child to learn that yes, language can indeed be confusing.

Avoid Sarcasm

Sarcasm is even more confusing than idioms. The intended meaning is the complete opposite of the literal words, and we rely on subtle inflections and the demeanor of the speaker to determine when sarcasm is being used and what its intended purpose is. Not surprisingly, nothing can muddy communication with an Autistic child more than sarcasm. Even neurotypical people sometimes miss its subtlety.

Avoid the use of sarcasm, either in words or tone of voice. Pay special attention to this accommodation if you're a person who uses a lot of sarcasm as part of your normal communication style.

Instead of rolling your eyes and saying:

👎 *You want to go to Disney World again this year? Oh sure! We have all the money in the world.*

Try just saying what you mean:

👍 *Disney World is fun, but big trips like that need to be planned. We need to save our money.*

If you find you have made a sarcastic remark, then hasten to explain yourself:

👍 *I was being sarcastic. That means I said the opposite of what I mean. What I really mean is...*

Some people bond through friendly, good-natured sarcasm. "You fumbled the ball again. You're really going to go far in this sport!" Please don't expect an Autistic child to do the social math on this kind of teasing. There is little chance that some Autistic children could even begin to decode the subtle inflections – *friendly, teasing, ironic, affectionate* – not to mention the contradiction of logic which literally states that fumbling the ball is a way to succeed. Oh sure, they're going to know EXACTLY what you mean. (Yes, I'm being sarcastic.)

Children on the spectrum *can* learn to recognize sarcasm. We want them to know about it, but I would not start with it. In families who bond through ironic forms of humor (where words and meanings go in opposite directions), the child may learn to recognize and use this form of humor, but how well will they handle it as they grow older? At best it's used for good-natured jokes, at worst (and perhaps more often) it's used to be mean to others. The difference is often in the eye (or should I say ear?) of the beholder. Will your child be misunderstood? Will your child know when *they* were misunderstood?

Autistic children need to understand sarcasm well enough to protect themselves from the mean form and avoid being seen as mean and obnoxious themselves.

Mark Up Your Language with Gestures

Think about all the important social cues conveyed by your facial expressions and tone of voice. *I'm joking. I'm surprised. I'm very concerned. I'm quite serious. I'm satisfied. I'm content. I'm delighted.* Can your child pick up on these cues, or does your communication style seem devoid of meaningful expression? It's not unlike the difficulties we all face when communicating in writing over the Internet. How many emails have been misunderstood because the intended tone of the communication was lost? Internet conventions try to address this problem by letting us mark up our written words with all sorts of visual cues such as the well-known smiley-face emoticon, abbreviations like "LOL" (laugh out loud), and other conventions that indicate our feelings and intent. Think of this when communicating with your child. How can you make your intent clearer?

You can use gestures to mark up your spoken words and minimize your child's need to read the more subtle social cues.

Let's start with the simplest of examples. Answering "Yes"? Then nod your head at the same time. Hold one thumb up, or two thumbs up for more emphasis. Answering "No"? Shake your head at the same time. Hold one or two thumbs down. Feeling neutral? Hold thumbs horizontally. These are standard, simple gestures. If you don't do so already, add them in when you are speaking.

You can go further. Exaggerate your expression and vocal tone. Smiling? Emphasize your smile with upward hand gestures at each side of your mouth. Frowning? Same idea: downward hand gestures will emphasize your frown. To convey sadness and sympathy, don't just say the words. "I'm sorry that happened" can be accompanied by your best sad face and a gesture on your cheek to indicate tears.

To validate your child's view that there is a BIG PROBLEM, spread your hands wide apart to emphasis the problem's size. Use an exaggerated facial expression that strongly shows your empathy and concern. "It looks like a BIG problem to me." And of course, use a matching tone of voice. This does not necessarily mean you should use a loud voice. Play with volume, speed, and intensity to see what works best. For example, if your child has sensitivity to sound, you can combine big gestures with a dramatic stage whisper.

Gestures make words less transitory. The word "happy" is here and gone in less than a second. A hand gesture lingers, pointing to your smile, giving your child a longer time to take it in, making communication more concrete and definite. This style of communication gives Autistic children a grounding point – a point of reference.

Abbreviate Your Language

Long phrases can be easily misunderstood by children on the spectrum. It's hard for them to know which words are the important ones. You can accommodate by using very abbreviated language. Avoid flooding your child with unnecessary information. Make yourself better understood by eliminating extra words. You are allowed to use incomplete sentences, but still use age-appropriate tone.

What words to eliminate? Prepositions, articles, and other connecting words can go. So, for example, "Ben, go and sit on the blue mat," becomes:

👍 *Ben sit blue mat.*

What else can we cut? Believe it or not, the noun "mat" might be unnecessary. Colors and shapes sometimes garner more of an Autistic child's attention than the names for objects, so we can simplify to:

👍 *Ben sit blue.*

You might be surprised at how well this works with some children. The technique came in handy at a recent gathering where I met Billy, an Autistic teen with minimal language, whose dad was trying to get him to pose for a photo with me. I observed as Dad repeated several times, "Billy, look at the camera," with no results. Billy was confused and distracted by all the activity around him. Fortunately the camera had a striking characteristic: it was bright pink.

"Billy look pink!" I said, and he immediately locked onto the camera, recognized its significance, and on his own said, "Cheese" with a big smile. His dad was more than a little surprised.

This example is not just about simplifying language. Language accommodations are tools that let us offer help at a deeper level. Notice how Billy needed help with focus. Once he knew where to put his attention, he tapped into prior experiences and knew exactly what to do. Honestly, I was a bit surprised myself when he said "Cheese" without any prompting. There was a lot more going on inside than was apparent by Billy's outer appearance.

When abbreviating your language, it seems an unusual choice to eliminate nouns and keep the adjectives. So what? If *blue* and *pink* speak louder to your child than *mat* or *camera*, you can use this insight to enhance your communication. Knowing how to adapt these accommodations is all about seeing things from your child's point of view.

This is not a natural way of talking, so it may take practice. I mainly use it with young children or when the child's verbal skills are not yet fully developed. Some children are fine with this style; others will notice the change and become uncomfortable. If your child seems distressed because you've changed your style of talking, then stop. Use this sort of "extreme abbreviation" at your discretion.

The general idea here is to match your communication style to your child's language processing ability. Don't pack too much information into one breath. Keep your ideas concise, and don't string a lot of unrelated thoughts together. Put space between ideas.

Also, avoid filler. It's too easy to fall into a stream-of-consciousness communication style, where important ideas are mixed in with idle chit-chat. This sort of style can be overwhelming to some children. At worst, it will stress them out. At best, they will tune you out. Take a breath between ideas!

Do you find yourself thinking out loud when communicating with your child? This is the style you want to avoid:

👎 *The hamburgers are almost done. Where's your father – is he still working in the garage? Oh my, what's that spot on the rug. Did you spill something? Oh, I remember now, that was there yesterday. Will you need help with your homework later? Where is your father?*

Stop and take a breath. Slow down your own thoughts. Which ideas are important? How is your child supposed to know? Perhaps all you really need to say is this:

👍 *Dinner is in five minutes. When dinner is done Dad can help with homework.*

Gauge what works best for your child. It may vary based on the relative calmness of the moment. If too much is going on, use shorter phrases to cut through the confusion. You might need to focus on just one idea. For example, focus on dinner or homework, not both. Yes, you can sequence multiple steps to make life predictable (Chapter 10), but in some cases it is best to focus only on the next step. Use repetition for emphasis:

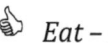

👍 *Eat – five minutes. Eat – five minutes.*

How would you support this with gestures? That's easy: a motion toward your mouth for "eat"; five fingers held up for "five minutes."

Some families are quite comfortable with a rapid-fire communication style. Maybe you were raised in such an environment. For many it is a way of bonding. Now here is a child who might not be able to keep up. Accommodate them. Shorten your sentences, focus your ideas, and take a breath now and then. That may be all it takes to keep a child from feeling like an outsider in their own home.

Using Metaphors to Connect

We hear that people on the autism spectrum are very literal, but we shouldn't take this stereotype too literally! Just because I recommend a literal style does not mean I believe that Autistic children cannot understand metaphors. Metaphors can help explain an idea based on your child's point of view.

Some children on the spectrum do very well with metaphors if you choose examples from topics that interest them. For a science-minded child you might explain feelings of liking and disliking others in terms of magnets that attract or repel. A child with knowledge of animals will probably relate to stories of animals who work together socially, versus those who hunt alone. You can raise a child's social awareness using metaphors – *if* you can come up with a metaphor that connects to their interests and applies to the situation at hand.

Language in Perspective

Language challenges are a part of autism, though not the heart of autism. Even if you fixed all the "superficial" language difficulties, you would still have issues underneath. It's important to keep this in mind as you learn to work out effective ways of communicating with a child on the autism spectrum.

For example, here is a logical statement that works well with some children but not others:

👍 *Please use a place mat because if you don't then the plate might scratch the table.*

For some children it is enough to explain why the mat should be used. Other children might not see the significance of a scratched table. It's not that they are uncaring or destructive; they just don't perceive why a scratched table is any sort of problem. They have no place to fit the extraneous information. In this case you need to add more:

👍 *If the table is scratched then I will be sad.*

It depends on the child.

As you reduce misunderstandings due to language, you will find yourself moving closer to your child's unique internal logic where they reach unexpected conclusions even when the information you have conveyed is perfectly understood. Language accommodations alone are not enough; still, they are important tools that will help you and your child move forward.

Have realistic expectations. When you have done all you can with language accommodations, there will still be challenges due to concept gaps and the emotional impact they cause. You might find it frustrating. Don't give up. We are by no means done working on language and communication, and throughout the book we will explore accommodations to go ever deeper. In the meantime, you can certainly overcome some communication problems with the techniques presented so far. I just don't want you to brush off a child's behavior as something solely due to a language disconnect. Most likely there is some combination of factors going on.

If we want to improve the quality of an Autistic child's life, then we need to understand the whole picture: language, logic, and emotions. Unfortunately I don't think that as a culture we've come close to doing this yet. I'd like to do nothing less than help change the way the world looks at autism. Is that an achievable goal? When I first wrote these words, my answer was that I simply didn't know. But time has passed as I've worked to get these ideas into print. Now I have hope. Change is in the air, and I'm not the only one who emphasizes the importance of understanding autism from the child's point of view. Maybe I can change the way *you* look at autism. That would be a big step forward.

Language processing is an important part of the picture, and it's the gateway to understanding those deeper issues. Improved communication bring insights into how your child's mind works. Become fascinated by it. This fascination has kept me going throughout my whole career.

5

Enter the Confusion Detective

Confusion is an ever-present thief, robbing your child of happiness. The worst thing about this thief is that he sneaks in right under your nose and steals something you might never notice is missing, until it is too late. Confusion steals your child's sense of safety and security. Confusion steals your child's trust in the world. Confusion steals your child's trust in *you*.

How does this thief get away with his bold crime? I'll tell you how: too few seem to know that he exists.

That's right. Confusion is too often overlooked, even when alarm bells should be sounding. Some parents miss it. "My child is very high functioning. He just doesn't have any friends." Some teachers miss it. "Zoey just acts that way because she has autism." Often behavior specialists don't even consider it. "David just wants attention. We'll come up with a behavior plan for that."

Everyone sees the symptoms; few are aware of the role confusion plays. As we've seen, language processing is one source of confusion. Sensory issues can certainly lead to confusion. Concept gaps can't help but lead to confusion – often extreme confusion. And extreme confusion leads to extreme emotions. When a child is having an emotional meltdown, everyone seems to wonder what has gone wrong. Amazingly, a critical clue is hiding in plain sight. The behavior itself should tell us that confusion is afoot.

How deep can the confusion go?

Jake had an extreme reaction when told the family would be going to the newly opened Mario's Brick Oven Pizza for lunch. Does he not like pizza? Is he staging a tantrum to get his way? Should this be chalked up to an inexplicable "autistic" reaction? These possibilities are suggested by a neurotypical viewpoint, but Jake's strong reaction tells us to look deeper. Maybe he is afraid of new restaurants. Many children on the spectrum are nervous about change; they find unfamiliar situations too confusing, so this is a reasonable guess. In Jake's case, though, the confusion went deeper still.

The unexpected truth emerged when his recent exposure to a certain electronic game came to light: it was a Mario game involving bricks. Could the similarity to the restaurant name have something to do with Jake's extreme reaction?

This actually turned out to be the case.

Perhaps Jake imagined walking into some strange or dangerous scenario from the game. Maybe he pictured Mario's bricks as pizza toppings. All we know for sure is that the whole idea of the restaurant made no sense to him. His image of the place was powerfully logical and unshakeable. He was being forced into a frighteningly bizarre situation, and his experience thus far in life gave him no assurance that anyone could keep him safe. Until the nature of his confusion was uncovered, nobody took his fear seriously.

People see emotional distress and unusual behaviors without ever suspecting their true cause because it can be hard to believe just how deep the confusion goes. I can't blame anyone for missing it. Just when I think I've seen every possible concept gap, a child will spring something new on me with a view of the world that I never considered before. This work is full of surprises.

How do we deal with it? *Expect* surprises! In any situation, assume there is an element of confusion until proven otherwise.

This sounds like the opposite of the "innocent until proven guilty" principle, but for children on the autism spectrum confusion is nearly always present. This is true whether you see it or not, so you must be on constant alert for it. And make no mistake: the child is not the only one who is confused. Misunderstandings go both ways. When confused adults try to help a confused child, what sort of result do you expect? No wonder some of the children I work with feel traumatized by those who have tried to help them.

Knowing that confusion is always present should bring some comfort, because now you have a concrete mission. In a very real sense

Enter the Confusion Detective

you have to become a Confusion Detective. Enter the scene as a master sleuth and try to spot the clues that everyone else has missed.

Okay, the image of Sherlock Holmes with his magnifying glass and deerstalker cap may seem to trivialize the problem, but I paint this picture to help you visualize your role. Confusion is a major issue, so I am quite serious about this confusion detective idea. We need to do something to help; we need to be willing to investigate every situation that arises. I absolutely think of myself as a confusion detective. I assume the confusion is there, and I begin to look for clues.

Neurotypical approaches often go wrong by ignoring the first clue: the child's own behavior. People are too quick to assume a neurotypical cause, or they simply label a behavior as abnormal and leave it at that. This unhelpful impulse sweeps aside important information. Instead, assume the behavior is a *normal* reaction to the child's experience, and you will begin to understand what that experience might be...*from the child's point of view*. Ask yourself: "What sort of experience would make *me* act this way?" It can be tricky because a child's conclusions about how to act will be based on conceptions of the world very different from yours.

Seeing yourself as a confusion detective is an accommodation on a grand scale, because it can motivate you to use all the other techniques that we're about add to your toolkit. At this point don't expect to have all the answers; just start asking the right questions in the right way. Think of the chapters ahead as pages from a detective's notebook with hard-won hints on how to do this.

Are you willing to be a confusion detective? I sometimes find it to be a lonely role, because so few seem to think such a thing is necessary. This general lack of awareness is one of the biggest obstacles we face when it comes to offering effective help for children on the autism spectrum. Compassion alone tells me we should be thinking outside the box, looking for creative ways to uncover each and every area of confusion. But there's a catch: if you're blind to the confusion, it's easy to ignore the need to look for it.

Always look for the confusion – your child's and your own. We need all the confusion detectives we can get. The more you see things through your child's eyes, the more you can expose this ever-present thief.

6

Facts Before Feelings

The ability to connect with others is a basic building block of human interaction. I want to be careful not to say that this building block is missing in a person with ASD. Certainly the *desire* to connect is there, but we can have such different perspectives that people (whether Autistic or neurotypical) fail to recognize the possibilities.

Connecting with an Autistic child is a bit like mixing Legos with Lincoln Logs. The pieces don't match, so it's challenging to build with them. Without a meaningful way to connect the pieces, everyone either gives up in the belief that it is not possible, or lurches forward without ever establishing an authentic connection.

And underneath it all, there's still a child.

Like me, you have no doubt seen adults successfully interact with neurotypical children too many times to count. A grandfather asks his 6-year-old granddaughter if she drove the car to visit him. She laughs and says, "That's silly," enjoying the joke. An adult steps in to help a child resolve a conflict in a kickball game; the child is grateful for the help. A sympathetic parent offers soothing words to a crying child, and the child soon calms down and explains what is wrong.

It is easy to imagine an adult connecting with a child.

Now what happens when these interactions just don't feel like connections? You try and your heart is in the right place, but the child does not respond in the way you expect. It's hard to interact with someone when it seems like a one-way street. Neither party feels good about it. It's sad, isn't it? Our natural neurotypical style suddenly does not feel so natural anymore when the child is on the autism spectrum. Our building blocks for communication don't fit. How do you joke around like grandpa? Or help resolve a disagreement in a game? How do you help comfort a child and dry the tears?

Here is my answer: begin with facts. Children on the spectrum want to connect. To reach them – and for them to reach us – we need lots of connecting pieces. Literal facts and logical information are comforting for Autistic children. These are some of the connecting pieces we are looking for.

Often Autistic children themselves will begin with facts to connect. In a restaurant one day a delightful young man turned around in his booth to talk to me. (This seems to happen to me a lot. I don't usually initiate these conversations, but I am more than happy to participate.) After proudly proclaiming he had autism, the teen began to give the middle names of various presidents, perhaps somewhat to the embarrassment of his family. He knew the 'B' in LBJ and the 'D' in Dwight D. Eisenhower, and explained that Harry S. Truman's middle initial didn't actually stand for anything.

His recitation of facts was all about connecting, so I stated a fact in return. "You know a lot about the president's middle names." And he replied that yes, he did. His keen interest in this singular topic – unusual as it was – offers a great opening to connect and understand him. To neurotypical people a barrage of facts can feel cold and off-putting, but they can be soothing to Autistic children. I think of facts as warm and fuzzy when I interact with people on the autism spectrum.

This chapter will present a number of accommodations based on the principle of putting facts before feelings. We can get to feelings by beginning with facts.

The Running Commentary Technique

What do I mean by *facts*? I am not necessarily talking about factual information which you might find in a trivia game, though I admit that having a better memory for this kind of information might make it just a little easier sometimes. I wish I had a better memory so I could recall all the facts and figures I learned in school and college. Alas, I don't. Still, I can relate by using facts. There are many different types of factual information in life. You don't need to know the distance to the sun or the president's middle name. You just need to make some

factual observations that seem to fit the moment.
Here are the basics of this technique:

Make observational comments. Even without a great memory for factual information, you can comment on what you see:

👍 *There are two cars in front of us at the red light.*

👍 *You are playing a video game.*

👍 *You are watching SpongeBob, and now there is a commercial.*

Do you see? These are observational comments. I call this the *running commentary technique* because you simply comment in a factual way on what is happening, as it happens.

Note the extremely literal approach. Weed out assumptions until you are left with the observation that seem least likely to clash with your child's view. For example, I would not assume a child with a stack of blocks sees it as a building or any other particular structure:

👍 *You have stacked up five blocks. That is good balancing!*

There are many other ways to use this technique. Here are some variations.

Compare and contrast. Just look for differences and similarities. No observation is too trivial.

👍 *You are drinking orange juice and I am drinking apple juice. We are both drinking juice.*

👍 *You have a pink shirt and I have a pink watch. We are both wearing pink.*

👍 *You are watching TV and I am listening to music on my iPod.*

Describe conflicts neutrally. State the simple facts, without any judgment.

👍 *You want to go to the movies and your sister wants to go to the playground.*

Label your own feelings. This helps with feeling recognition.

👍 *There is traffic. There are many cars going slowly on the road. I wish we could be going faster. I am frustrated.*

Slip in some social information. Some facts may seem too basic to consider sharing. Share them anyway:

👍 *Most people don't like waiting in traffic.*

Don't assume that every child knows this! You can point out the illogical nature of the situation if you think your child will see the humor in it:

👍 *Nobody likes to wait in traffic. Isn't it strange that so many people are doing it?*

This sort of "illogical logic" can spark a discussion and bring in the laughter for some older children. That in itself is pretty wonderful, if and when it happens. As a bonus, you get to slip in more social information:

👍 *People sometimes have to do things that they don't like.*

Explain the behavior of others. Your child might be confused by the behavior of others; it helps to explain. This is an opportunity to teach social information without focusing on your child's own behavior.

👍 *Sally is standing up because she has difficulty sitting still.*

Help your child see the positive in other people. Looking for the positive goes deeper into explaining the behavior and intentions of others, and puts in some groundwork for discussing your child's own behavior in a validating and constructive way.

👍 *Alyssa is using a loud voice, but her words are very nice.*

Communicating with facts takes a bit of getting used to. You'll become motivated when you see how well it works. It's just a habit that most people don't develop because it's not usually needed for neurotypical communication. Get in the habit of observing and sharing facts. The running commentary technique is a great way of using facts to connect and move things forward.

Comments Before Questions

When a child is crying and nobody knows why, adults hasten to find an answer. "Use your words," we say. "Tell me what happened. I need to know why you are crying so I can help." The child is gently questioned about what is wrong. The questions show we care. The child tells their story and is comforted, and everyone feels better as the problem solving begins.

However, this approach can be very scary to a child who is on the autism spectrum. Our typical questions about what is bothering them are intended to bring comfort, yet some clients of mine have said it actually makes things worse. The reason should not be a big surprise: problem solving about emotional issues requires a great deal of social know-how, which is *not* an area of comfort for children on the spectrum. Therefore, addressing a problem with direct inquiries often inflames the discomfort – very much the opposite of our intended outcome.

Even before you know what the problem is, you can help by starting with facts. Facts provide comfort. I know, it's not so comforting for the adults; we want to get to the bottom of the issue as soon as possible. But impatience pushes the possible further away. To achieve our goal, and especially to avoid creating a new problem, we need to have the utmost patience and be willing to try another approach.

Make literal observations. It is often hard for Autistic children to identify and express feelings in a way others understand. It is a source of stress for them. I try to avoid words like *upset, sad,* or *unhappy*. Instead, I use literal observations:

👍 *There are tears on your face. It looks like there is a problem.*

These words are crafted for a child who has difficulty identifying emotions. A literal fact (tears on your face) can make communication more accessible to such a child, providing an opening for them to be heard and understood.

Give opportunities for a child to correct you. I liberally add these kinds of "outs" to my statements:

👍 *I think I am right, but I could be wrong.*

A literal observation is not very comforting if it does not match the child's point of view.

Offer reassurance. When giving social information that might sound critical, make sure you mix in positives so that your child stays open to the information.

👍 *You are not in trouble, but I have some important information that you might not know. If you take crayons at school without asking, people might think you are stealing and not borrowing. I know you would not steal anything, because you're very nice.*

Make validating statements. Be both validating and *normalizing*.

👍 *Problems are really not fun. But they do happen sometimes.*

This lets a child know that problems are a normal thing in the world and that having a problem does not mean you're strange or peculiar. It's about acceptance. It's quite acceptable to have a problem to solve.

Giving facts like this will often calm a child down. It is a moment of connection. Notice that you still don't know what the problem is. We just have to accept that we usually cannot calm the child *and* get the information in a single step, hence the need to break the process down. Factual comments are comforting. Questions are not.

* * *

I have chosen my words carefully in these examples. I deliberately avoid referring to emotions until I am sure a child can identify with the words and is not intimidated or stressed by a discussion of their feelings. It may sound like an unusual way of speaking, but this fact-based approach eliminates one more stress point when working with certain children. It is very helpful to find the right "literal level" of language that is appropriate for the individual child.

Give Concrete Choices

Finally, we come to the point of asking a question. Open-ended questions can be hard for a child who does not understand the context. It can be too overwhelming for them to figure out what information is required. Give concrete choices when asking questions.

Instead of saying, "How was school today?" try questions like these:

👍 *Was your school day good, bad, or in the middle?*

👍 *Did anything new or interesting happen at school today?*

👍 *Do you remember seeing Bob in school today, yes or no?*

This accommodation works well for casual, everyday conversation. It helps your child feel comfortable giving specific information that you might not learn when your questions are too general.

The accommodation can also help a child with decision making. Instead of saying, "What would you like for lunch," give some options:

👍 *For lunch would you like soup or chicken fingers?*

The Connection Formula

Concrete choices are especially important when your child seems distressed. Begin by putting comments before questions (*it looks like there is a problem, problems are really not fun...*). Is your child calming down? Do you have their attention? You may need to wait a few minutes before asking questions.

When your child seems attentive, offer concrete choices:

👍 *Is this a small problem, a medium problem, or a BIG problem?*

👍 *Did the problem happen before recess or after recess or during recess? Or was the whole day a problem?*

The goal is not to immediately solve a problem; it is to start a conversation and keep it going. The path to problem solving begins by getting the problem on the table, as we will see in the second part of the book.

> **Keep the Conversation Going**
>
> Conversation is a social interaction, and if you can keep the conversation going in a way your child enjoys, then you are giving them valuable socialization experience. A subtle but important goal is to make the conversation feel worthwhile to your child. You need to prove the value of the social interaction, and gauge how well you have done in this regard.
>
> The longer a child is willing to engage with me, the more evidence there is that I have proven my worth at some level. From that point I can start to lead the interaction. Someone looking on might not realize what I'm doing. They will see me making jokes, being silly, and talking about unimportant matters. Well, that is in fact what I am doing. I enjoy it, and here is the point: *so does the child*. And that is why it's so important.
>
> Think of it this way: It is hard to lead if no one is following. But once you have the ability to lead, then you have the groundwork for the more advanced steps to come.
>
> Trying to start a conversation with a child on the autism spectrum is hardly a new idea. However, people who recognize

its importance often pummel the child with questions in order to get them talking. That is a natural inclination; it is *not* what I aim for. You don't need to keep the conversation going at all costs. A child should *want* to talk and interact. I want children to be motivated to interact. In the beginning we do not necessarily try to lead. Yes, you will be eager to convey helpful social information, but for now it is enough just to keep the social connection alive and well for as long as you can without creating discomfort or anxiety in your child.

As you ease into asking concrete-choice questions, there's one choice that is always important to offer...

"I don't know" Is an Okay Answer

When a child answers "I don't know," how do you interpret their answer? For me it depends on whether or not they are on the autism spectrum. For some neurotypical teens, "I dunno" is a stock answer for everything. It conveys a sense of aloofness, as if they can't be bothered to answer you.

For children on the spectrum, answering questions is an entirely different matter. Any of the following situations might be possible (and you can probably think of more):

➢ They don't understand the words or idioms that were used to phrase the question.

➢ They don't understand the context of the question.

➢ They misunderstand both words and context, then struggle to answer a question you didn't really ask.

➢ They are confused or disoriented by the question. Even questions of preference (*what would you like for lunch?*) are difficult for someone who doesn't know how to go through the decision making process.

➢ They know the answer but can't find the words to express it.

> They would ordinarily know the answer but are feeling too much pressure and their mind is racing.

> They're afraid of answering wrong.

> They don't understand the relevance or importance of the question. "Where does it hurt?" may rank with "What is your favorite color?"

> Their focus is elsewhere; the question didn't get their attention.

> They don't know that questions are meant to be answered.

> They literally just don't know the answer.

In most of the scenarios above, it is reassuring to the child if they know they can say, "I don't know." It takes the pressure off. You will usually want to make "I don't know" one of your concrete choices.

I find this accommodation to be so helpful that I post it in socialization group rooms as one of the rules. It's right there on the rules list, which the children themselves helped to create. *Rule #12: I don't know is an okay answer.*

I can tell you that it's a very comforting rule for some of the children, because it is mainly a rule for adults. Group leaders are required to accept "I don't know" as an answer. Of course we're allowed to rephrase our questions as needed; for example, by offering more concrete choices. Or we may change the topic and approach it later from a different direction. It's important to be aware of the child's emotional readiness for a conversation, and back off when things get too stressful. "I don't know" is the child's safety net.

Some parents find "I don't know" to be a disrespectful answer, and think I will somehow spoil a child by not holding them accountable. This is neurotypical thinking for neurotypical children. I assure you that I do set limits. I just want to first make sure that the child understands the concept behind each limit, otherwise they can feel defeated by an endless list of rules to memorize.

Another neurotypical view is that the child thinks an honest answer will get them in trouble. And they could be right...but do they know *why*? A neurotypical child will usually know exactly what they did wrong. Can the same be said for a child on the spectrum? The very concept of "trouble" might have its own unexpected definition in their view. For example, I have known Autistic children who hold themselves to an impossible standard. Did you ever struggle and fail to perfectly express your feelings on a topic? A child might actually feel like they are telling a lie if they can't find the perfect words. Someone like this might go silent when questioned on a topic, even if you're only making small talk. Then again, a child might correctly understand that they really are in trouble, yet still be totally in the dark about the reason. For some, trouble has no reason. They might know only that behavior X produces punishment Y with no deeper awareness of the connection. Discipline can seem very random to a child on the spectrum, making them extremely cautious as a matter of self-preservation. You need some very reliable communication to uncover these concept gaps. It takes time.

I'll let a child off the hook if that's what it takes for them to feel emotionally safe. I prefer "I don't know" to frozen silence. It keeps the conversation going. My goal is to gradually hand accountability over to a child, but first I have to know their conceptual readiness. In other words, I need to know how much they don't know. If your child doesn't have an answer (even if you think they should), please make it safe for them to tell you so.

The True or False Game

True or false are the quintessential concrete choices. Making a game of them serves a few purposes. It helps make a child comfortable with conversations on difficult topics; it gives you insight into how your child thinks and feels; and most importantly, it allows a child to feel comfortable talking to you. Remember that social interactions are hard for children on the spectrum, and this includes talking to parents and other adults – especially adults with lots of confusing questions.

Initially play this game just for fun. Explain to your child that you're going to ask some questions and that they can answer *true* or *false*. Yes, do let them know that it's also okay to answer *I don't know*.

Start with easy questions such as:

👍 *True or false: You like chocolate?*

Most children know whether or not they like chocolate. If it happens that they don't know, then "I don't know" is a great answer too, as it keeps the game alive.

To keep things light, ask a few questions that are comically false. For example, if it's a really hot summer day then I might ask a question like this:

👍 *True or false: It's snowing outside?*

I do this because it's stress-free and generally kind of funny.

You can allow your child to take turns asking their own questions if they want to. When the questions are humorous, there can be a lot of laughter as you each try to top the other's silliness. When the mood is light, you can sometimes angle toward more important questions. If it proves too difficult for your child, retreat back toward humor.

I once ran a dating workshop for Autistic teens. They were anticipating a topic that would be confusing and hard for them to understand. To break the tension I was a little silly, asking questions like, "True or false: I have three heads; I have four noses; there is a giant bird in my hair..." etc. I knew the members of the workshop very well, and they were certainly familiar with my silly humor. We had fun with this for a while, then I asked, "True or false: You want to date?"

The majority of the participants responded with "I don't' know," and that in itself was very helpful information. With the mood still light, we were able to dig more deeply into their concerns.

Provide some fun ways for your child to give their answers. They can answer verbally, write their answer on a piece of paper or tabletop whiteboard, point to an answer that is already written down, choose a flash card with the answer on it, etc. When we play this game in a socialization group, the clinician writes the words, *true, false* and *I don't know* on three different whiteboards around the room. Then a question is asked, and each child goes to the whiteboard corresponding to their answer.

This "game" is actually an effective technique that allows you to probe for important information. It is best not to come on too strong, as if interrogating your child on the witness stand. Try to be laid back during the activity. Play it cool! You want them to be open and willing to interact, so it's best to take it slow and have fun. Add in more serious questions a little at a time. In other words, wear your detective hat but don't "spook the witness." Resist the urge to push for too much information too soon.

After all, you are just a parent who wants to have a good connection with your child.

> **Picking Just One Toy**
>
> A family was getting ready to go to a neighborhood barbeque. The parents told their three children to pick one toy each to bring with them to the event to keep themselves entertained. Two of the children picked out their toys within minutes and were ready to go. The third child, an 8-year-old boy on the autism spectrum, was found sitting in his bedroom, crying with his new activity book in his lap. Was this his choice, or was selecting just one toy an impossible task?
>
> His parents asked some True or False questions to find out.
>
> "True or false...You picked your activity book?" Yes, the boy said. That was true. A good choice, thought Mom and Dad. He could occupy himself for a long time tracing mazes and solving puzzles in the book.
>
> "True or false...You want to bring another toy, too?" Also true. Wisely, Mom and Dad avoided any recrimination in the question, so their son would know he was not in trouble for wanting to bring a second toy. The game helps you stick to facts and tread gently when near sensitive feelings.
>
> "True or false...The other toy is your Nintendo game?" No, this was false.
>
> The guessing game could have continued for some time, but the boy was a lot calmer now, so Mom just came out and asked.
>
> "True or false...You can name the other toy that you want to bring." The boy nodded: *True*. He would name the other toy. And he held up his pencil.
>
> This is how the boy's parents learned that he viewed the activity book and the pencil as two different toys.

I highly recommend using this activity both for fun and to learn how your child perceives situations. It's a way to ensure accurate communication. Teach it as an enjoyable game before using it for more serious matters. Please, do *not* use it as a way to find out who spilled grape juice on the sofa. Protect its value to your child. The *true or false* game is worth playing just for the shared moments it can bring.

Feeling Phrases

A school behavior specialist once made this insightful remark regarding children on the autism spectrum: "The more language a student has, the more opportunity there is for misunderstandings and confusion." Although that statement sounds self-contradictory, in my own practice I have found it to be all too true.

When a child has strong language skills, many assume there is a comparable degree of social understanding. Often the opposite is true. A child might be adept at using language in such a way that it masks their misunderstandings. (It can be quite unconscious on the child's part, since they, too, are likely unaware that a misunderstanding exists.) This irony easily misleads parents and professionals alike, producing an even more confused child on a downward emotional spiral. The number of misunderstandings throughout the day cannot be underestimated.

Lindsey was a middle school student on the autism spectrum who invited everyone in her English class to her birthday party. Not one of them responded to her invitation. A sensitive teacher approached her, and Lindsey agreed to speak with the school psychologist. After telling the psychologist she was not upset, Lindsey left the office, took a pair of scissors from the secretary's desk, and stabbed herself in the hand.

She ended up as a client of mine.

Although academically exceptional, Lindsey did not know what words like *sad*, *disappointed* and *upset* meant. Oh, she knew the dictionary definitions. She simply didn't relate them to feelings within herself or understand their relevance to her situation. Strong verbal ability is not the same as emotional awareness. Autistic children tend to think in literal, concrete terms. Feelings, though, are extremely abstract. Without the right tools, miscommunication is inevitable.

Facts Before Feelings

Fortunately, there is a way to use concrete language to identify feelings: associate something concrete with an emotion. For example, if a family once had a fun trip to Disneyland, you might ask, "Are you Disneyland happy?" Of course if Disneyland was over-stimulating and stressful, you could use it as an expression for those feelings, for example: *Disneyland stressed*.

I call these *feeling phrases*. They are simple phrases that associate something concrete with an emotion.

A boy is afraid of thunderstorms, and you are quite familiar with his level of anxiety when a storm is brewing. When faced with a new social situation, you ask:

👍 *Are you thunderstorm scared? Are you more scared than when there's a thunderstorm, or less scared?*

A girl becomes mad when a page in her book rips. The next time she gets mad, ask:

👍 *Do you feel like 'ripped book' mad? Are you more mad than ripped book, or less mad than ripped book?*

Lindsey and I did a great deal of work along these lines, in effect creating a personal dictionary of concrete terms, a sort of shorthand for feelings. "Do you feel disappointed like the time your video game broke?" became simply: "Do you feel *broken-game*?"

Using a few expressions like this, we were able to establish a common language whereby she could express her fear and disappointment. As it turned out, she felt overwhelmed not only about this one incident; she pretty much felt that way about most of her school day. She was relieved to have someone validate her feelings and also take action on them. I'm happy to report that Lindsey has come a long way. She has changed schools and now has a group of authentic friends.

Feeling phrases were not the only accommodation I used, but it's an important tool that not only helped us adults get to the heart of Lindsey's feelings, they helped her feel understood and significantly less afraid of life. At last she had some allies who could help her feel safe. Do you get the idea?

The Connection Formula

Remember, feeling phrases should always be based on past events where the child's emotions have been accurately identified:

👍 *Do you feel 'new puppy excited' about vacation at the beach?*

New puppy excited works only if a child was truly excited when the new puppy arrived. For some children, *new puppy nervous* might come from that experience. The more emotions you can correctly identify, the more you can build your personal dictionary.

You don't always need to include a "real" word for an emotion in a feeling phrase:

👍 *Do you feel 'illogical homework' like from Miss Smith?*

There might not even be any conventional words to describe the feeling of 'illogical homework.' The meaning will nonetheless be vivid to a child who has experienced it.

In the beginning, using a neurotypical label is less important than giving your child a way to express themselves. Lindsey certainly knew what I meant when I asked "Do you feel *broken-game?*" Feeling phrases gave us a yardstick for comparing and contrasting her emotional experiences – and more importantly, it gave her the concept that such a thing is even possible.

* * *

How many of these phrases do you need? Just one or two to begin with. Usually you'll need to come up with them yourself and try them out with your child. Some children are able to pick their own phrases for different feelings, often using lines from TV shows or movies – a good reason not to be dismissive when they tell you about their favorite character for what seems like the millionth time. They are giving you a vocabulary. Make good use of it.

It is not always easy to know if you have the right phrase associated with the corresponding feeling. It takes trial and error to see if your child responds emotionally in a way that matches your assumptions. And conversely, your child will be looking for a response from you that matches their view of things. Support communication with gestures and facial expressions to make your own responses clear. The conversation has to make sense to both of you.

One way to verify a feeling phrase is to use another one of the accommodations. For example if a child says *broken-game* to express their feelings, give concrete choices in a follow-up question:

👍 *Is that a small, medium, or big problem, or don't you know?*

If it is a small problem, then you might be able to let it go. If you find out it is a BIG problem, then you can add "broken-game" to your feeling phrase dictionary. And don't forget to validate your child:

👍 *Oh, so it's a BIG problem. Nobody likes big problems. We will have to solve it.*

Some children will independently modify their expressions as they mature, using standard ways to express their feelings more directly. They will prefer to use conventional words (*happy, sad, frustrated, disappointed*) once they know how these relate to their experience.

Use feeling phrases along with other accommodations to steadily build more reliable communication with your child.

Find Connecting Logic

A child on the autism spectrum will need our help to understand the neurotypical world in a way that lets them enjoy life. We can offer them a new perspective, but we will need to prove its validity. Frankly, we will not be able to prove anything unless we can help the child understand our viewpoint in a way that is logical to their way of thinking. Our logic must relate to something the child has experienced or can imagine experiencing.

Let's say that Cody always likes to go to cash register #7 at the supermarket. It is something familiar – an anchor point. Perhaps there is a snack there that he likes. Register #7 has always been open each time Cody has been there. One day register #7 is closed. Cody is disoriented. How can we help him understand? Try to logically connect the situation to things he is familiar with. See if you can you spot the connecting logic in the following:

The Connection Formula

👍 *The cashier at #7 is not there. Maybe she is home sick. Maybe she is on vacation. It is not normal for #7 to be closed. The person at #5 is not sick or on vacation. He is here today. Both #5 and #7 are odd numbers, so they have something in common.*

If you feel the last statement about odd numbers contains the connecting logic, well of course you're right. In fact, *all* of the details above relate to connecting logic. Cody has experienced everything that is mentioned: being home sick, being on vacation, and of course the feeling of something being "not normal" about the whole situation, at least from his point of view. (Remember, even though in your experience register #7 has probably been closed on many occasions, for Cody, this is a first.) So everything in this example is intended to connect in some logical way to Cody's own experiences and viewpoint.

You can use any kind of connecting observation:

👍 *The person at #5 has a yellow shirt. You have a yellow shirt.*

👍 *#5 has gum, #7 has corn chips. They are different, but they both have cash registers.*

All of these logical connections set the stage to convey some social information:

👍 *If you really want chips from #7, you can get them and bring them to #5. The manager allows you to do this. I am 100% sure it is okay.*

Does this all seem a bit much to you? It's a very concrete and logical way of talking, and it does sound strange when you're not used to it, especially when you hear the tone of voice that I use – sometimes very animated, other times very matter-of-fact. I adjust to find what the child responds to. When I do workshops, audience members have actually laughed when they hear me demonstrate this way of talking. Someone once asked me, "Do you *really* talk like this?"

My answer: "You ain't seen nothing yet."

Yes, this very literal and logical style sounds peculiar when presented out of context. Very few people are instantly comfortable adjusting their way of communicating. At the same time, one of my most frequent questions comes from parents who hear me talk to their children: "How did you know what to say, and how can I learn that?"

If you're motivated, you will learn. If you see results, you will have no problem building on this technique.

Practice finding the connecting logic. Make your conversation concrete and logical. Notice we are *not* directly addressing Cody's feelings, nor are we dismissing his feelings. We are not saying: *Get over it. This should not upset you.* Quite the opposite – we allow him to feel okay about having the feelings he has, and we gently try to broaden his horizons by finding connecting logic as a starting point.

> **Soothing with Logic**
>
> Connecting logic is a way to provide relatable explanations for situations that appear random and scary to a child on the spectrum. It's a very helpful soothing technique. When your logic relates to what your child has already experienced, then the situation appears more normal to them, and your child is better able to manage their feelings about it.
>
> When you use this technique, you are also planting a seed. Many children on the spectrum can learn to learn to self-soothe with logic when you lead by example.

Basics Before Social Skills

Let's say that your child is often agitated when they come home from school. You suspect there is an ongoing problem, and don't know what it is. How will you get to the bottom of it? You wish your child would simply talk about their school day and tell you what is so upsetting. You press with questions, and that triggers an even stronger emotional reaction.

This is a fairly typical scenario in which parents expect a child to have not only the coping skills to discuss a problem, but also the basic building blocks to recognize that there even *is* a problem. If a child is not able to understand and identify their own feelings – much less connect them to the source (such as a situation at school) – then the parent's questions are irrelevant and confusing and will often just make things worse.

Neurotypical thinking is focused on traditional social skills, and barely considers all the basics that must be in place for a child to respond to a simple query such as the following:

> 👎 *Did something happen at school today? You seem upset. Why don't you tell me what is upsetting you?*

Is this really such a difficult line of questioning? Well, what sort of response do you get? It can vary greatly.

➢ Does the child know what it is to *seem upset*?

➢ Do they think this is a quiz with a right and wrong answer?

➢ Do they think they're in trouble?

➢ Do they expect to be punished if they don't answer correctly?

If we could see beneath the surface, we might understand how disconnected our line of questioning is from the child's reality. We might find language confusion. There is usually anxiety. The child might not even understand the context of the conversation. You could be asking them to connect an emotion they can't identify to an event they can't pinpoint through a chain of cause and effect they can't perceive, all while they feel threatened by the possibility of punishment. And so we get silence, or a shrug, or a strange disconnected response. Or a meltdown.

With some children we get an answer like this: "Of course things happened at school. How could things not happen at school?"

Under the surface all of the emotional confusion and anxiety is there, but this child simply has no way to recognize or articulate it. Since the emotional component of the question makes no sense, we get a perfectly logical response that to us sounds disrespectful. I hope you see it isn't meant that way.

If you're lucky, you get a "disrespectful" response instead of shrugs and silence. At least it's a conversation starter, *if* you are willing to connect with their logic:

👍 *Yes, you are right. It would be very strange if nothing at all ever happened at school. My words were asking a very strange question. I see your point of view. My question was not very logical.*

In a case where a child simply can't respond, I truly wonder what is going on inside. Perhaps they are thinking without thoughts, experiencing a wordless ball of bad feelings that they must escape for survival. If they could express the bad feelings, we might hear:

Not safe not safe not safe not safe not safe not safe not safe...

I do not wish to overdramatize this scenario, but I assure you I have worked with many children whose anxiety has frozen them into silence. Now tell me, for a child who is in this *not safe* place, what relevance do traditional social skills have? We need to begin at a much more basic level. If a child literally cannot parse the meaning of your words, is this the time to teach about responding promptly when an adult asks a question? If a child answers in a literal way (*Of course things happened at school today...*), should you take offense and teach about showing respect? When stress pushes children into an emotional meltdown, should you label them as "bad" and dole out the punishments? No, no, and absolutely *no*.

The idea of punishing a child for their neurological difficulties horrifies me beyond words. Yet this is exactly the approach that is often applied to Autistic children. A child is utterly confused by an adult and is unable to respond in the expected manner, so the adult goes in a direction that is even more incomprehensible. The two are worlds apart and growing further apart by the minute.

This child needs a lifeline, not a lecture.

Remember, all we wanted to do was understand a child who might have had a problem at school so we can begin the problem solving process. There are many practical ways to do so without pushing them further away. We now have a lot of tools for this kind of situation . Let's apply some appropriate accommodations:

The Connection Formula

Put comments before questions	"On weekends you look happy, but after school you do not look happy. It looks like there could be a problem, but I could be wrong."
Offer reassurance	"You are not in trouble, but I am going to ask about school..."
Give concrete choices	"How are you feeling? Good, bad, or in the middle? 'I don't know' is an okay answer."
Use gestures and animated speech	"I have some VERY important and INTERESTING information to give you..." (I'll have more to say about labeling important information in Chapter 15.)
Normalize your child's feelings	"Did you know people can have very different feelings on the days they go to school and the days they don't go to school? It is normal to have different levels of happiness at different times."
Use feeling phrases	"Was your day better than 'lost homework' day or worse than 'lost homework' day?"

Do you see how we use the accommodations to comfort and connect? Although we have not yet found the cause of the problem, we are building the trust that will be needed before proceeding. We are throwing out a lifeline.

7

A Child's Lifeline

A study in 2013 found that children with ASD are far more likely to consider suicide than neurotypical children. Twice as likely? Ten times more likely? If only. According to the study, published in *Research in Autism Spectrum Disorders, Volume 7, Issue 1,* Autistic children are 28 times more likely to think of taking their own lives.

While I don't wish to dwell on scary statistics, I do want you to understand that I am absolutely serious about the needs of these children. Too many will need rescuing when it is close to too late.

What does it mean to be a child's lifeline? I have a very simple definition: you are someone who helps them feel safe and understood.

Fear of Feelings

Many Autistic children have difficulty self-soothing, and that in itself can be very scary. Imagine being a child with emotional discomfort and not being able to calm yourself. You might not realize that parents and other adults have the role of helping you; their efforts to soothe you make things even scarier. Adults don't understand what's wrong, you don't understand their ways, and so it does not feel safe to trust their efforts. You are left to your own devices.

Can you see why even the very idea of emotions becomes fearsome to some children? With no tools to regulate and self-soothe, a child becomes more and more afraid of their own feelings, like a runaway train. In order to help children on the spectrum understand and process emotions, we need to offer the type of help that they are open to receiving.

Accommodations offer a lifeline in a way that will feel like *real* help to your child. I know that you are trying hard to connect, that you desperately want your child to feel safe and understood. In order to accomplish this, your child needs to be motivated to follow your lead. The techniques you have been learning are geared towards this goal. Accommodations get you close enough to your child for them to accept the tools you have to offer. Then you will be able to guide, nurture, and parent your child towards social independence.

> **Gentler Ways**
>
> By the way, please refrain from directly asking a child if they feel safe and understood. It is a complicated question and could be very confusing. As you have been learning, there are gentler ways of approaching questions about feelings.
>
> As you start to see life through your child's eyes – and as they sense your sincere effort and growing understanding – then both of you will learn from each other and find ways to share how you perceive things.

Looking for a Superhero

A number of years ago I stepped into the hallway outside my office to meet Art, an Autistic boy I would be seeing for the first time. As I greeted his dad, I spotted Art engaged in a little bit of acrobatics involving a stairway railing. In the blink of an eye he swung around and let himself go, to land ungracefully at his dad's feet. Though unhurt (there was thick carpeting on the stairs and floor), he was understandably shaken. His reaction: he jumped up and ran around the hallway, flapping his hands, calling out words that at first I couldn't quite make out. It was an emotional meltdown all too familiar to the dad, who quietly told me in a concerned manner, "He does this often, saying things that make no sense."

"Well, seemingly," I said. But my inner detective was already trying to figure it out.

What word was Art repeating, and why? I started with the assumption that it did make sense somehow, and was not just a random word. In this case I got lucky. Art's dad was holding a Spider-Man book. The

A Child's Lifeline

words clicked. Art was calling out the superhero's nickname: "Spidey! Spidey! Spidey!"

I inquired about the book, and learned that Spider-Man was Art's favorite superhero. What if Art was calling his hero for help after that frightening fall? My instincts told me to try this assumption.

"Dad is Spidey," I said to Art.

At my prompting, Dad played along. "That's right, I'm Spider-Man. I can help."

What effect did this have? Well I should warn you that I might have guessed wrong; my words might have disrupted Art's reality. Perhaps Art had imagined *himself* as Spider-Man during his acrobatic misadventure, and would be disoriented when I switched the role to his dad. An unexpected association can trigger an emotional meltdown in a sensitive child. However, when you're already dealing with a meltdown, there is less at risk. In this case it just seemed likely that Art was calling a familiar and comforting name. As it happened, I was right, or at least close enough. Art went to his dad and calmed down immediately.

When it works – when you make a connection to an Autistic child – the result can be almost magical. I don't want to oversimplify; it can take a lot of work to get to this point. In this case I slipped into my detective mode, took in a few clues, and got lucky with a reasonable guess.

The shift into this mode of thinking can be a big adjustment indeed. I'm happy to say that after this one small success, Art's dad made the adjustment rather enthusiastically, and has found many more ways to connect with his son and help him feel safe and understood.

Your child almost certainly won't express their needs in a neurotypical way. In their world they might be looking for a superhero. Can you see yourself in that light? Please don't think it is a silly idea. You have to wear The Connection Formula like a superhero's mantle. It has to be part of you.

8

Make Problems Visible

Blake had an unusual way of showing he was nervous: a smile was his typical response to anxiety and confusing situations. His true feelings were not readily apparent. School personnel said to me, "He's fine, don't worry about it." Then at school one day, with a smile on his face, he deliberately hit his head against the wall.

This can be a difficult possibility to accept, that you simply do not know what your child is feeling. You may think you know – you may be absolutely certain that you know – and still you may be wrong. Even professionals misinterpret the outer signs.

In this case the professionals blamed the family, openly stating that the parents must be abusive. In truth, school was simply too stressful, and Blake was doing everything he could to keep it together for as long as possible. This sort of situation is very serious. Being under this amount of stress on a daily basis is unacceptable. It can lead to serious mental health issues, including significant anxiety and depression. It is not okay to let it continue.

What can be done?

I have already described some ways to improve communication. With some visual accommodations, we can do even more.

As the name suggests, visual accommodations add something concrete and visible to your interactions. This includes drawings, printed pictures, charts and graphs, physical objects – anything that helps make communication more tangible and real.

Many Autistic children are visual learners. Broadly speaking, visual learners understand and process information better when it is given, well, visually. It helps when they can see it. A visual representation lasts longer than the spoken word. That's why I use gestures and exaggerated facial expressions to support the spoken word.

Communication is deliberate and focused when done visually. And, when we enhance communication with visual elements, it makes it easier for someone on the autism spectrum to understand our intent.

Please keep in mind that this is not about simply adding visual support to a neurotypical communication style. Instead, use visual accommodations in conjunction with The Connection Formula principles; it's a style that comforts and connects. Use language accommodations, avoiding idioms and sarcasm. Put facts before feelings. Give concrete choices. And now, add in some visual elements. Part of helping a child feel safe and understood involves helping them understand you. The other part, of course, is finding ways to understand them. The visual accommodations in this chapter can help you understand each other.

Visual 1-5 Scales

For Blake, visual 1-5 scales worked well to uncover his stress level. Blake's face did not reveal his feelings, nor could he express how he felt in words. Yet he could point to a number on a visual scale to show that he felt nervous or scared.

I've shown how concrete choices help a child know what to focus on. Visual scales build on this idea by showing the choices using simple graphics. A 1-5 scale is a visual way for a child to express how they are feeling on a scale of one to five, where five represents the most intense feeling, like the pain scale that a doctor might use when he asks you how much something hurts. These types of scales are also used as rating scales in questionnaires. Here they are used in a slightly different application. For our purposes, it is very helpful to have a physical copy of the scale printed or drawn on a sheet of paper. It's a way to make feelings visible and concrete.

Such a visual representation of emotions is easier than language for some children, and once your child is familiar and comfortable with problem scales, the process of using them can calm things down in stressful situations.

Let's look at some variations and learn the best ways to use them.

Make Problems Visible

The Safety Scale

The 1-5 scales can be used with a variety of topics. I call this one a "safety scale" because it helps the child express how safe they feel. (Color versions of all the scales can be viewed on the website given on the title page. The color darkens to red on the right side of the scale.)

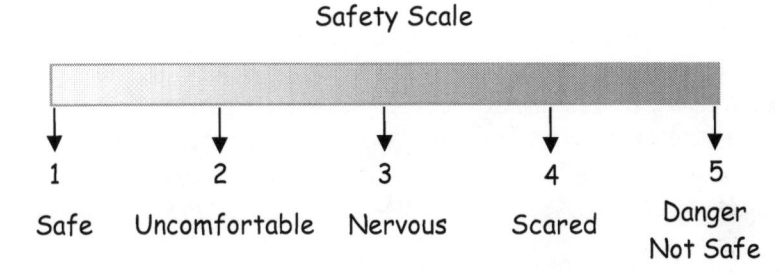

Safety Scale

1	2	3	4	5
Safe	Uncomfortable	Nervous	Scared	Danger Not Safe

Here is how I described this scale to Blake. You can vary the explanation to suit your child.

1. **Safe**: You feel comfortable and do not feel stress. You are not worried about your body or your feelings getting hurt. You do not have any fear.
2. **Uncomfortable**: You can handle the situation, but you have a little worry. You think the worry will go away soon.
3. **Nervous:** Fear is becoming big enough so you notice it and you want it t go away. You try to stop the nervous feeling, but when you try it doesn't work. Your feelings may be a little hurt, but your body is safe.
4. **Scared**: Your body or feelings do not feel safe. Something needs to change as soon as possible. Your feelings are very strong in a bad way. Something is definitely wrong!
5. **Danger:** This is an emergency situation! Help is needed now! Your body and feelings could get very hurt.

Ask your child to point to the level of safety they are feeling regarding a particular situation. I have used this scale not only to ascertain how a child is feeling, but also to teach different levels of safety. Some children are not attuned to safety – they can be unaware that they're in an unsafe situation. It's a concept gap that needs to be bridged, and the safety scale helps.

For teens in high school I have explained that when someone asks you to do something and you don't know what their words mean, then don't agree to do it. I explain that this is an unsafe situation, and that it makes me nervous – a level three on the scale. Anytime you reach a level three or above on the safety scale, it's time to take action.

By the way, it won't do to introduce this scale for the first time during a crisis. In a moment I'll give you some tips for introducing the scales to your child. First, let's see a few more variations.

The Logic Scale

Rules and social conventions just don't seem logical to a lot of the children I work with. (Honestly, some social conventions don't always make sense to me either, but I realize their value in allowing me to connect with the world around me.) If a social convention doesn't make sense to a child on the autism spectrum, there is a good chance they won't follow it.

The logic scale is extremely helpful to learn what makes sense to children on the spectrum. Use this variation of the 1-5 scale to discover how your child perceives social conventions, such as the rule to raise your hand in class or the need to take turns talking. You might be surprised by what you learn.

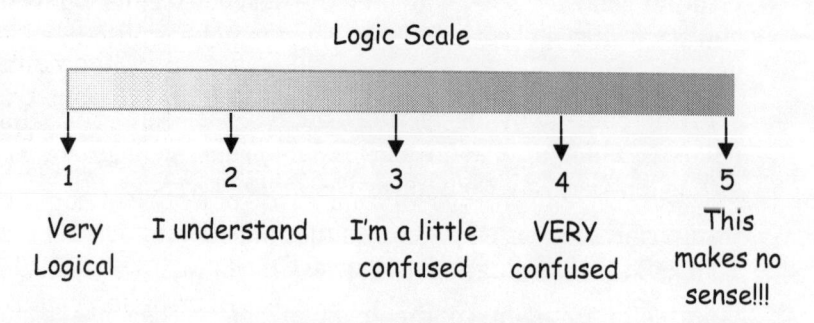

Logic Scale

1	2	3	4	5
Very Logical	I understand	I'm a little confused	VERY confused	This makes no sense!!!

Always remember, this is for *you* to see from your child's point of view. This is *not* to tell them how logical they seem to us.

Make Problems Visible

The Feeling Scale

A 1-5 scale can easily be used in conjunction with feeling phrases (Chapter 6). These use your child's own experiences to label their feelings. Say you want to rank these feelings from one to five:

1. Very happy
2. Happy
3. Neutral
4. Sad
5. VERY sad

Here is a feeling scale that might work for some children:

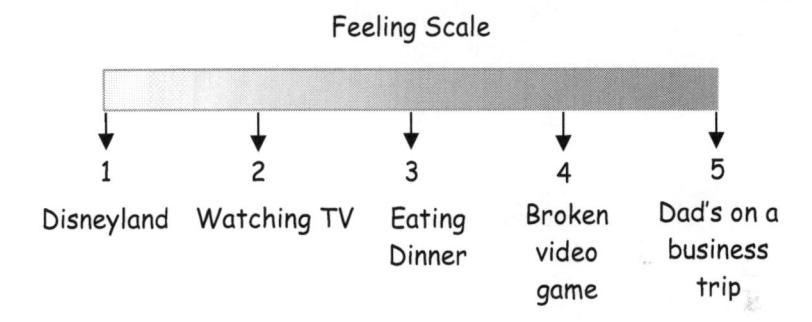

Feeling Scale

1	2	3	4	5
Disneyland	Watching TV	Eating Dinner	Broken video game	Dad's on a business trip

A scale like this can help assess how a child feels about a particular situation by comparing it to experiences from the past. Adapt the scale to your child's perspective. Does dinner really belong in the neutral center of the scale? Certainly not for all children. What about tying shoes? Feeding the cat? Math homework? Bedtime? Letting your child rate things on a feeling scale might spark some interesting discussions...*if* your child is into the idea. (The rating activity itself might not rate very high, and that, too, is good to know.)

The more you use the 1-5 scales to learn about how your child views various activities and situations, the more information you have for creating new scales. And the more you learn about your child.

It's certainly a way to keep the conversation going.

The Connection Formula

Introducing the Scales to Your Child

It is best to introduce a 1-5 scale when your child is calm and relaxed. Do not wait for a crisis to bring up the idea for the first time. If a child is feeling overwhelmed, it will just be too much of a bombardment to their senses. They won't know why you are introducing this new thing, and you could end up confusing them and associating bad feelings with the scales. Instead, introduce a scale when things are going smoothly.

Start with questions that are not emotionally charged for your child, and make it a game for the whole family. Bring out the scale and ask everybody, "Show me on the scale how you feel when you're watching your favorite TV show." You can participate in this yourself by pointing to how you feel in the situation.

If and when your child becomes accustomed to the scale (this may take days or weeks), you can ease into slightly more serious questions, like "How do you feel when someone in school breaks a rule?" Again, give your own answer. If a situation does not apply to you, talk about when you were younger or imagine how someone else you know might respond. Just be careful not to ask too many probing follow-up questions in a row. Tread lightly.

Once a child is comfortable with a 1-5 scale, they might begin to use it on their own initiative. It becomes a wonderful self-advocacy skill that can help both child and adult know when to take action. It is obviously important for adults to know that a child is hurting emotionally long before things reach a crisis level.

Problem Scale Variations

It is helpful to have a variety of 1-5 scales available to cross-check what you learn using other accommodations. Over time you want to provide as many tools as possible to help your child identify and express feelings on their own. This can be very difficult for Autistic children, so it cannot be pushed too quickly. In general, it does become easier each time you are able to use an accommodation to slow things down and get things right.

Do the scales have to go from one to five? No, although it's a good place to start, especially if your child is not used to any other system. I

Make Problems Visible

have heard of teachers who insisted on a different scheme (say, a 1-10 scale) even when the child was already familiar with the 1-5 system. Why on earth would a neurotypical adult be rigid about this? Inflexibility is the opposite of accommodation. If your child prefers a different scale, work with it. Let them start at zero instead of one, or count backwards, or completely forget about numbers and use colors or letters or animals. Your goal is connection and communication. Flexibility is the key. Try lots of ideas until one of them works, then refine and change as you and your child move forward.

The website given on the title page has a few other problem scale variations, and includes some blank scales for you to copy and use. Or feel free to make your own. You can draw them by hand or use whatever computer software you might be familiar with. I made mine using PowerPoint.

The Problem Pyramid

The problem pyramid is a variation that represents the size of a problem. Larger problems are represented by larger segments in the diagram. At the very top, all is well. The biggest problem is at the base.

Use the example on the next page as a starting point to create your own, or print the color example from the website.

> **Checking Your Work**
>
> One purpose of the problem pyramid is to "check your work" by using it in tandem with other accommodations to make sure communication is clear.
>
> When learning arithmetic you were probably taught to check your work. (I was taught this way.) So if you were asked to subtract 20 from 120 and got 100, you would then add 100 + 20 to make sure you got back to 120. In the same way, you can use a problem pyramid to double-check information learned from a 1-5 scale. If the results agree, you can move forward with more confidence in the information.

As you surely know, it is hard to figure out exactly what is wrong when a child on the spectrum has a problem. If you do not understand

The Connection Formula

the nature of the problem – and especially if you're not even aware that a problem exists – then it's impossible to develop a solution which your child will be able to understand and accept. Problem scales help you and your child make the problem visible.

The Problem Pyramid

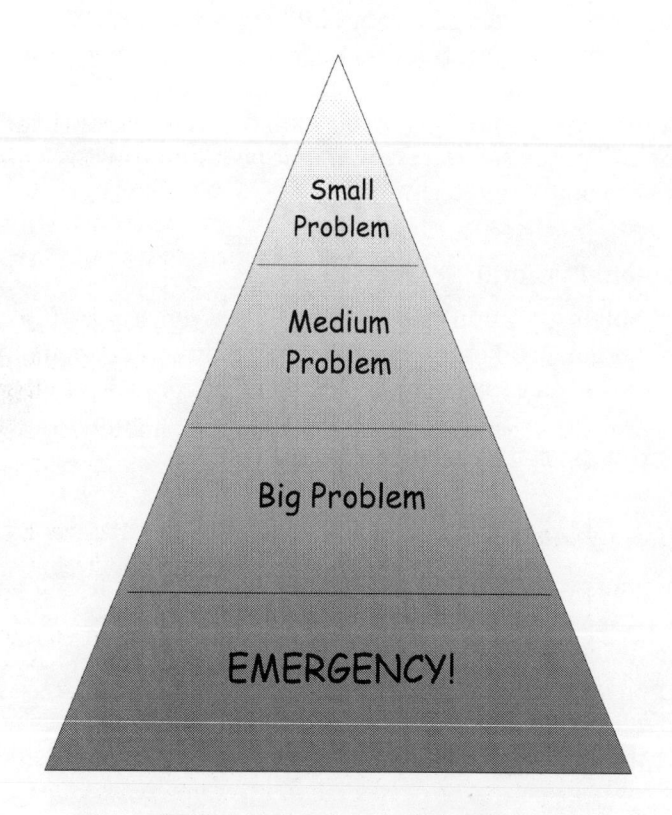

- Small Problem
- Medium Problem
- Big Problem
- EMERGENCY!

How big is your problem?

Point to the size of your problem, or put a checkmark on your problem size.

9

Change Is a Nightmare

Children on the autism spectrum often don't know what to attend to or how to prioritize what they observe in their environment. It's a real source of stress in daily life, as the following story illustrates.

A mother sent her son into a bakery to pick up an item she'd ordered. He had been there many times, but this was the first time he went in alone. After a few minutes, he returned to the car empty-handed and explained that the bakery had been rebuilt. When Mom went in to investigate, she found the place as it had always been, although unusually crowded, with people standing in front of the take-a-number dispenser, blocking it from easy view. Because he did not see the familiar dispenser, her son thought the shop had been rebuilt. His mother could not convince him otherwise.

This type of experience leads to a loss of confidence. The world appears to be a crazy and random place, disorienting and overwhelming. If situations like this are not handled sensitively, the child will be at risk for more serious emotional difficulties. It's easier to understand a child's anxieties and unusual behaviors when you realize how differently they perceive the environment.

Trauma and Loss

Whether it's a rearranged classroom, a substitute teacher, or juice served in the wrong colored cup, change for Autistic children can indeed be overwhelming, confusing, and even earth-shattering. I believe in many cases we are seeing the impact of trauma and loss.

Lest you think I am overstating the problem, allow me to fill you in on a bit of my background. Over the years I have worked with many neurotypical clients. When counseling teenagers who were depressed and suicidal due to trauma such as sexual assault, and when working with younger children who had experienced difficult losses, I found that some of their symptoms were similar to those exhibited by Autistic children – children whose backgrounds, on the surface, did not suggest they had suffered any such extreme experiences.

Could it be that for an Autistic child, daily living is a traumatizing experience in and of itself? Over the years I have sadly confirmed that yes, Autistic children can suffer an extreme sense of loss because they do not feel safe in a confusing world that makes no effort to accommodate or understand them. This is not only a trauma of the past – it is an ongoing experience. For all too many Autistic children, trauma and loss are part of the daily routine.

I hope you can begin to imagine the enormity of this situation.

The Disappointment Ratio

Have you noticed that your sense of loss is generally proportional to your level of anticipation? If somebody else ate the last cookie, your disappointment is rather small in the scheme of things. On the other hand, if you'd practiced all your life for an Olympic gymnastic performance only to fall off the balance beam at the critical moment, then the sense of loss will affect you much more deeply. We all suffer disappointments large and small, and our emotional response is normally in sync with the size of the event.

This is all rather intuitive and obvious. So why do I point it out? It's because the ratio of anticipation to disappointment does not always work this way for Autistic children. More correctly, the ratio works, but on a much different scale. You might say that our "compassion meters" are not calibrated to detect the deep sense of betrayal that a child might feel over even the slightest disappointment or change of plans. A fairly inconsequential inconvenience to you might be crushing to the child. Any young child might cry when told they can't have that ice cream cone before dinner; neurotypical children get over it quickly. However, an Autistic child can experience it as a profound loss – as if ice cream itself and the very concept of all happy things have been removed from the world forever. We know otherwise, so we don't take the child's reaction very seriously.

Even knowing the possibility of this extreme perception of loss, it is hard not to brush it off as unimportant, merely a temporary disappointment. Of course ice cream will continue to exist! But that's not the point. The point is that the child is suffering an emotional wound that will not be retroactively healed by their next treat. In other words, the perception is wrong, but the wound is real.

Complicating matters, consider how hard it is for some children to self-soothe. The experience of strong emotions is wounding in and of itself. This doubles the stakes for such a child. Their long-term trust in life, and in themselves, is not as easily restored as an ice cream cone.

For some children, life is lived on that Olympic balance beam, and any breeze can knock them off. The sense of loss and confusion may be so great that it can take weeks, months, or longer to heal the damage. Yet in so many cases, before the healing can even begin, they are knocked off balance once again. And we, the neurotypical adults in their lives, seem to have no idea what's going on. It just doesn't make sense to us. We say that their emotions are out of proportion to the experience, but we are judging the child's experience based on what it would mean to *us*, not them. And so this concept gap between us produces that other gap I have mentioned: the compassion gap.

Recalibrate Your Compassion Meter

I start with the premise that the child's emotional reaction connects in some logical way to their experience. This gives me a sense of how extreme the experience might be, and helps me go to the core of the problem in order to comfort, connect, and begin a healing process. What I've discovered is that Autistic children experience untold losses every day. It's as if the present moment is the sole focus of their life. When they do not get what they expect in the moment, it may feel like it will never happen. It's not just about a specific loss such as skipping a treat or losing a game or missing a favorite TV show; it's about living in a world that is not predictable or safe. It's about not having the tools to self-soothe and navigate change. It's about chaos versus order.

When anything in an Autistic child's life goes awry, the feeling of disappointment can be huge. Imagine training for that Olympic moment. Then, when it is your turn, you are told that you cannot perform. No sensible reason is given, and everyone acts as if it's no big deal. In tears, you seek help. You ask your coach, your parents, the game officials. They look at you without a glimmer of understanding and say, "Calm down, you are overreacting."

You and I both know that in this situation the feeling of disappointment and confusion would be overwhelming. A strong emotional reaction is quite understandable considering the scale of this colossal loss and unfair treatment.

Now we have two things to consider for a child on the autism spectrum. First, the child may feel an extreme level of disappointment and confusion, even for changes you might consider minor. Second, the child may have concept gaps related to emotions and difficulties with emotional regulation. For such a child, strong emotions arise when unexpected changes make the world feel untrustworthy, and then the problem is compounded by panic over the emotions themselves. The panic becomes part of the loss.

Regardless of the triggering event, the loss is very real—it is not imagined. For the child it is just as big a loss as it is for that Olympic athlete. This is not a matter of being spoiled or thin-skinned. Please adjust your approach accordingly. The next time an Autistic child in your life displays a strong emotional reaction, recognize it as a valuable window. They are showing you their emotional reality. Imagine the scale of their loss, and consider how *you* would react. This alone will guide you to a better way to connect.

The long term effect of repeated loss and disappointment... of being told you are overreacting...of not feeling safe and understood...is significant, and saddens me very deeply. A pat explanation (*he is crying because he's Autistic*) does not erase the reality behind a child's emotions. The trauma is real. Recalibrate your compassion meter and you will see.

10

Make Life Predictable

A good many Autistic children do not fully understand the nature of linear time. Cause and effect, beginning, middle and end – consider how life would feel if these concepts were missing. A child might not understand the need to plan and make choices, as if we all can do exactly what we want right now. A carefree life? Well, the darker side is that such a child can feel buffeted by arbitrary events beyond their control and comprehension. How would they know when things are going to happen or why they're going to happen?

Life can seem very random for children who have difficulties with time, and randomness can be scary. Have you ever watched a scary movie? Some people like the thrill of a good scare, when you don't know what is around the next corner and wonder what will jump out of the dark. But even if you like to be scared at the movies, you wouldn't want to have that feeling every day, all day, now would you? Never knowing what to expect leads to emotional vulnerability, and this is the reason why it's important to work on the concept of time with Autistic children.

For a child who is afraid of the next random event, we need accommodations that shine some light into the darkness. We need to make life predictable.

Sequencing Life with Visual Schedules

If the concept of time is problematic, so is the concept of a schedule. Learning about schedules is feasible for some Autistic children, and they are open to the concept. Others need to make peace with the idea.

But the imposition of a schedule makes certain children feel like they are being robbed of their life. From the outside such a view is very hard to understand, and so we miss the need to explain that schedules are there to prevent time from slipping away before we accomplish what we want. Many children do understand the reason for schedules, yet have unreasonable expectations of just how much control a schedule actually gives them. They might not realize that a schedule cannot change the steady flow of time or force everything to happen when we want it to.

Whether you are planning a vacation or simply preparing your child for a routine day, it is helpful to give them factual information about the plan. Sequencing the information puts it in a logical order so your child can understand what to expect:

> *We will go on vacation to Grandma's house in three days. When it is the day before vacation, I will help you decide what toys to bring. We will then put the toys in this box before you go to bed. The next morning we will get up early and pack the car. I will help you put the toy box in the car.*

Sequencing gives structure and makes life feel less random. It is calming and comforting. But are words enough? Talk is here and gone. Time is fleeting, and so is the spoken word, whereas a visual schedule is tangible and permanent. It's a reference point. A child can look at a visual schedule and feel comforted to know what will happen next.

<u>Written Schedules</u>

Let's start with a written schedule. I often use portable whiteboards for these. You can also create one on a computer and print it out. I number the items and include a check box. Many children enjoy checking off each item after it has been completed.

- ☐ 1 - Eat breakfast
- ☐ 2 - Get dressed
- ☐ 3 - Thirty minutes of screen time
- ☐ 4 - Go to the zoo

Make Life Predictable

- ☐ 5- Look at animals for one hour and then eat lunch
- ☐ 6- Maybe look at more animals or go home

Depending on the needs of your child, you might need to break things down into specific steps; for example, just the breakfast routine:

- ☐ 1 - Sit at the kitchen table at 7:00am
- ☐ 2 - Tell Mom the cereal you want: Cheerios or Rice Chex
- ☐ 3 - Mom will pour cereal in your bowl and you can watch
- ☐ 4 - Mom will pour milk over the cereal and you can watch
- ☐ 5 - Use your favorite blue spoon to eat your cereal

Note that I included the exact time. For some children, you might want to add the word *approximately*, then explain:

👍 *It is better to be early than late. Mom can wait an extra minute to pour the cereal, but the school bus will not wait.*

There is a lot of social information hidden in little details like this.

Pocket Schedules

A pocket schedule uses photos or representative items placed in pockets such as those found in hanging shoe organizers. The pockets are large enough to fit items such as crayons or small toys. Clear pockets are best because they make it easy to see the items.

I sometimes use doll furniture and other toys to represent an activity on the schedule. It is important for the item to represent the activity as clearly and obviously as possible. For example, what could be more obvious than a toothbrush to show when it is time to brush teeth? You might even pair it with a small tube of toothpaste. I have often used plastic food from toy kitchens to represent a mealtime food. The more something represents the actual activity, the better. In a pinch you can use simple line drawings, but try to think beyond this. A photograph is clearer than a line drawing, and a physical item (if available) is more tangible than a photograph. I have also used scrapbooking 3D stickers. They are slightly raised representations of a wide variety of day-to-day events. Think creatively! It's usually not necessary to use the same type of item in each pocket; I use toys in some and photos in others. You can see a photo of a sample pocket schedule at the website given on the title page.

Pocket schedules are excellent for young children or for those who have difficulty understanding the concept of a routine. They make the social information more accessible.

> **Making Routines Concrete**
>
> Some children on the spectrum have difficulty remembering certain routines. The child's logic and priorities don't connect up with the steps we want them to follow. Just because a routine is obvious to you, don't assume it is obvious to your child.
>
> For example, putting on shoes first while still in pajamas will make getting dressed rather complicated. This makes perfect sense to you, but does it make sense to your child? There is a definite logic to the procedure of getting dressed, and the logic here might be easy to demonstrate, and therefore easy for your child to remember.
>
> The logic of other routines is harder to explain; for example, washing hands after using the bathroom. The idea of germs might be very hard to demonstrate. If the logic isn't clear, the routine will not be clear. Even though it doesn't clarify the logic, a schedule helps to make the existence of the routine more obvious. Make the routine as concrete as possible and you will have a head start on clarifying expectations for your child. This helps reduce confusion.
>
> Is logic alone enough to help your child remember the routine, or do you need some sort of schedule? It's good to have a variety of options available.

Photo Schedules and Guides

Visual schedules and guides can be created using a variety of photos kept on a computer and arranged as needed to fit the planned activities. You can lay out the photos in a grid or on a timeline, or make a slideshow with them.

As a counselor, I sometimes email photo guides to parents so their children will know what to expect at my office. I include a picture of the entrance, the rooms they will see, and the staff they will meet. Schools can likewise share photo guides. Due to current technology these are becoming easier and easier to make. They don't need to be printed; a child can look at them on a computer or phone.

Talking Picture Schedules

Today there are many smart phone and computer applications that you can use to make a talking picture schedule. (It took me just a few minutes to figure out how to do this using PowerPoint.) Sequence the pictures, and record a brief description to go with each one. Now each picture has a caption your child can hear. You can even let your child record their own voice into the schedule.

Silent Timers

Keeping track of time is something that everyone does on a day-to-day basis – and it is another challenge for some children on the spectrum. I like to use a large timer – something that is easy for the whole family to see during timed activities. A Time Timer® is ideal – these clearly show "how much longer" without hard-to-read numbers. They come in a variety of sizes and allow the whole family to see, at a glance, how much time is left. And this is especially helpful: these timers make no sound. You can be aware of time without the distraction (and pressure) of a ticking clock.

Introducing the Idea

Many parents have asked me how to introduce a visual schedule. Here is what I do:

First I explain to the child that almost all adults use calendars or appointment books. This normalizes the idea. Show that schedules are a normal part of life. If your child questions you about schedules when you first introduce the idea, be sure to explain that almost all adults use them. We also use grocery lists, to-do lists, etc. It is a very natural thing to do. Teachers certainly use schedules as part of their curriculum planning. Your child might like to hear about that!

I might show a child the calendar on my computer or phone. This gives them a concrete reference point so they know that schedules really are used by everyone and are not unusual or strange. "Lots of people have schedules like these," I explain. I use a very matter-of-fact tone of voice and don't make a big deal out of it. Then I explain that it is helpful for children to know what is planned on the schedule. After all, why should adults be the only ones who know what the plans are?

Because I am low-key and matter-of-fact, I typically have success. If you are concerned that your child might be resistant to the idea then you can quietly post your own schedule on the refrigerator or in another obvious place. As your child gets used to seeing you use it, it will become a more familiar process and they will probably become more open to it.

You can expect a few different reactions when you introduce schedules. These are some things to be prepared for.

Rigidness about timing. Your child might want to know the exact timing of things. Many children become concerned if they don't get to all the scheduled items on the specified day or at the specified time. If you are not going to get to an item that is important to your child, then make a future plan for the activity, and be specific. If you're not sure about the specifics, then *make a plan to make a plan*. (That's an important problem solving strategy discussed in Chapter 16.)

If the activity is very important then you can promise it will happen. Please, keep track of your promises! You can write them down in a "promise notebook." A child can feel a sense of loss when time runs out for a favorite activity. A promise notebook helps to minimize your child's feeling of loss, but of course you need to build a track record of reliable follow-through.

Rigidness about changes. Some children believe that if an item is on the schedule, then it must happen or the rules have been broken, which feels unacceptable – even if they were not particularly looking forward to the activity. I often explain that we don't need to get to everything on the schedule *this* time, and there is more time in the future to do things.

The child changes the schedule. In some cases a child may erase or cross out an item that they don't want to do. At least they are communicating! This gives you the opportunity to explain why it is on the schedule. If possible, let them reorganize the sequencing of events.

On the other hand, more than one child has added time to my timer when they are enjoying an activity. They don't want it to end so soon. Some do it in a playful way; others might believe that they have really turned back time, which leads to some interesting problem solving when it becomes apparent that it didn't work. Handle this sensitively. Allow more time if you can, though that is not always possible. Remind your child that there is more time in the future.

The Sequential Walkthrough

If I asked you, "Tell me everything about your work day today..." you might hesitate, wondering where to begin. On the other hand, if I were to ask very specific questions, like a detective, it would give you a starting point for your recollections. "Was the light red or green when you reached the corner of your street this morning? Was there traffic when you got onto the highway? Where did you park when you got to work? Was it hard to find a parking spot?" Do you see how these questions bring concrete images to mind?

A neurotypical person may find it easy to select some significant highlights from the day without this kind of detailed prompting, whereas an Autistic child might not know what is important to report. Their day could be a blur of memories zooming by like a rewinding video recording. Or the child might have a single-minded focus on some small detail to the exclusion of all others. We're usually not going to know their exact experience. Even so, I have found that a sequential walkthrough can help children get "unstuck" when they don't know how to answer a question. It's a good way of offering concrete choices. The child does not need to figure out what is important and what is not. That is the job of the detective: you.

The general idea is to take things in sequential order: *Getting on the*

The Connection Formula

bus, arriving at school, going into class, going out for recess, taking the math quiz. However, the point is *not* to ask a bunch of rapid-fire questions. (You don't want to come off *that* much like a detective!) The objective is to find a conversational path that is specific and has information your child can relate to. For example, you can begin by doing a walkthrough of your own day. Note how this example includes some connecting logic:

👍 *After you got on the bus today I got in the car and drove to the grocery store. I was on Park Street going to the store and you were on the bus going in the other direction to school. That's interesting to me. We were both on the same street at the same time.*

Observe your child and see if they are paying attention. Do they seem comfortable, or are they looking at you like you're an alien? Maybe they are annoyed or have tuned you out. If so, then change your tactics. You can still stay with the walkthrough and just change it up a little, or you can switch to a different accommodation.

Your child might make a comment related to the grocery store, the street, or the school. Even if your child doesn't chime in, that's all right. As long as they are mildly interested and comfortable you are in good shape and can continue talking.

👍 *My end of Park Street was sunny with a few clouds. How was the weather on your end of Park Street? Was it sunny too?*

Giving these types of parameters will make it easier for your child to join in the conversation. Remember to include your child's interests:

👍 *I did not notice any airplanes in the sky. Did you?*

It is always nice to walk through your respective days and compare and contrast just for the fun of it.

Now we have an approach for asking your child about their day in school. "How was your day?" is just too general, so we take things in chronological order. Sequence from one thing to another; back up and reverse the sequence if you'd like. The main idea is to think about the different parts of your child's day to give the conversation a focus. Remember to put comments before questions. Start by giving facts.

👍 *Today is Tuesday and I remember that on Tuesdays you have music. Is my memory correct?*

If your child says "yes," then you can add:

👍 *Thanks, I was just asking because usually your memory is much better than mine.*

If your child says no, you can say:

👍 *Oh, that's my mistake. My memory was wrong!*

As you focus on each part of your child's day, ask specific questions with concrete choices:

👍 *During music class, did you practice that song the class will be doing for the assembly next week, did you do something else, or both? It's okay if you don't remember.*

Hopefully you will get a response here. If so, make a comment that relates to their response, and then move on.

👍 *After music class it is lunchtime. I made your favorite sandwich for lunch today. I try to make it the same way each time. Did I make it the same way or did I add too much almond butter?*

I like to throw in some humor now and then, so if the sandwich was a hit, this could be the time for some silliness. The idea of having a conversation can be stressful to Autistic children. Jokes bring an upside. Associate a little fun with the difficult challenge of small talk.

👍 *Oh good, I'm glad you liked the sandwich because it would be really strange if I made a mistake and put the almond butter on the outside* of the bread. That would be hard to eat! I would need to add lots of napkins. If I put the jam on the outside too, then that would be a VERY messy sandwich!

Ideally by now your child will be laughing and trying to figure out how one would eat such a sandwich. This could create an interesting conversation! Now that the ice is broken, go on to ask more about lunch.

👍 *Did you notice anything interesting during lunch? Did anyone have inside-out sandwiches? Did the teachers wear their clothes backwards? Was it a normal lunchtime, or did something different happen? Did anything extremely 'not fun' happen? Things out of the ordinary are very interesting to me. Things that are really fun or really 'not fun' also interest me.*

Notice that the number of questions has increased, but many of them are silly questions. This pairs the idea of questions with the possibility of fun. By keeping it light, you can angle toward more information about the day. Your child might tell you about other events at lunch, or simply say that nothing very interesting happened. If these conversations remain fun, you may learn more the next day.

Because it imposes a natural structure, a sequential walkthrough forces you to break down information in a logical way, helping you make sense to a logic-focused child. Think of it as a framework for organizing facts and information. The purpose is simply to interact with your child in a manner that is not off-putting to them or uncomfortable for either of you.

A walkthrough does not have to use strict chronological order. You can jump around on the timeline:

👍 *Thanks for telling me about lunch. Before lunch you have social studies...if my memory is right. I don't know why they call it social studies. Do you?*

Your child might say "no" or give a nice explanation. Either way, you can validate the response and then gather some more information:

👍 *I wonder what the teacher did in social studies today. Do you happen to remember if she used the whiteboard? Or did you read books, watch a video, or do something else?*

If your child is interested you can continue asking questions. If not, then quickly and calmly change the subject. The goal is twofold. You want to learn about your child's day so you can help them navigate through school. You also want them to be comfortable talking with you about school...and about pretty much everything else. It's a way to start a conversation and keep it going.

Sequencing with Rating Scales

To gain further insights, you can combine a walkthrough with a 1-5 scale to learn how your child feels about events. Where does the Social Studies class rate on the logic scale? Does lunchtime feel safe?

You are not limited to the past. You can combine the 1-5 scales with a sequential walkthrough to anticipate the future.

Here's an example. Bruce, who would be starting Middle School in the fall, began to grow irritable during the summer. When asked if anything was wrong he would always say, "No." Now as I've mentioned, you can't always get reliable answers by asking so directly. Despite his answer to the contrary, Bruce's irritability was a sign of anxiety, and his concerned parents wanted to pinpoint its source.

There was one clue: Occasionally Bruce would mention that he didn't like the color of the new school, suggestive of negative feelings about it. Some anxiety about the new school would be quite natural, but it's always good to get confirmation and assess the degree of concern.

When Bruce's parents told me about this I encouraged them to use the 1-5 Safety Scale. Bruce and I had used the scale many times in my office, so I knew he was comfortable with it. I instructed his parents on how to approach it, reminding them to deal with Bruce's feelings in a matter-of-fact manner so as not to add any new stress on top of whatever he might be feeling. I also told them how to apply the idea of sequencing to a future event: an imaginary walkthrough of the first day of school.

From their account I'd say they did a good job. In an everyday tone of voice they walked their son through this scenario: "When you wake up on the first day of school you can have your favorite cereal for breakfast. Please point to the 1-5 scale and show me the safety number." He indicated 1: Calm. They went on to lead him through the morning: getting into the car, driving to the school. All calm.

These walkthroughs can vary greatly. Some children may indicate a 3 or higher right from the first step; others might need to be led right to the specific scenario that concerns them (finding the right classroom, meeting a new teacher, going to recess for the first time, etc.).

Bruce's parents got to the part about arriving at the school. "When we get to the Middle School, I will drop you off at the front door, by the crosswalk near the yellow buses." Bruce pointed to 5: Danger – Not Safe! Then he told his parents he wanted to stop the game.

Bruce's parents concluded that he must have a great deal of anxiety about the new school. His answer on the safety scale (and his reaction to the "game") had made it pretty obvious. They were correct, of course, and we were able to deal with this in therapy over the summer.

> **True Support**
>
> It's important to note that I'm referring to a clinical diagnosis of anxiety. This was not a case of back-to-school jitters – that's looking at the situation through neurotypical glasses. A neurotypical child will have some coping skills, including the ability to identify the source of their nervousness, the ability to self-sooth, and the ability to work through their concerns with the help of friends and supportive parents.
>
> Bruce lacked these abilities, so even though he had very supportive parents, it would have meant very little if they did not have a way to translate their support into reliable communication, and then translate what they learned into action.

For Bruce, the prospect of starting at the new school felt like being dropped into a jungle with no coping skills. It was not as if he didn't know what to expect; in a way, he knew all too well. He expected confusion and danger. The neurotypical response: *Oh, don't worry, everything will be okay.* That is not a plausible claim for someone whose new school experiences have never been okay before. Fortunately Bruce's parents were now on top of things. They put many accommodations in place over the summer: A visit to the school; photos of teachers; a picture schedule showing classrooms; a plan to call home during the first day.

Summer preparation also included more sequential walkthroughs, which grew more detailed as Bruce was now able to visualize stepping through the school door without triggering a level five safety alert. We were now walking through hypothetical situations, and for any contingency Bruce could think of, a plan was put in place. As his therapist, I thought of a few contingencies of my own. Arrangements were made for Bruce to check-in with the school counselor periodically during his first day, and these check points became part of the plan. The walkthrough turned into a schedule of sorts, a schedule that was comforting to Bruce. I'm all for over-planning. This plan for Bruce made his life predictable.

Sequential walkthroughs are very versatile. They work for the past and they work for the future. You can use them to identify a source of concern, and you can use them to make schedules and plan for contingencies.

Every child is different. Accommodations can be used in many combinations. The way in which you and your child work with them becomes part of your mutual dictionary. Reliable communication means *reciprocal* communication. As we move forward, we want your child to seek you out as someone who understands them, and as someone who they understand.

Part 2: Preparation

Connect Before Correct

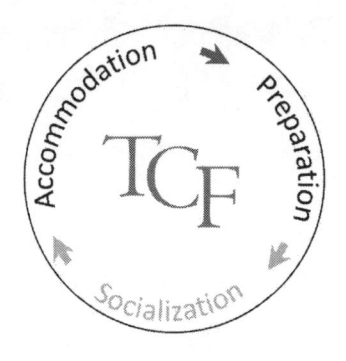

We want to motivate your child. We don't want them to feel beat up by the process. We don't want them to feel constantly wrong. We want them to feel connected.

11

Conceptual Readiness

Someone once asked me, "What is the one biggest difference between Autistic and neurotypical children?" I could not come up with a concise answer in the moment because the differences are so vast and varied. Perhaps the best answer is this: if you saw the world through an Autistic child's eyes, you might not recognize it.

Most people see obvious differences in behavior and that all-too-common difficulty socializing. Few, though, suspect the true nature of the differences, or how profound the real differences are.

I have used the term *concept gap* to refer to the deep conceptual differences behind the superficial view. Revelations about a child's way of thinking can leave professionals surprised and parents shaken. Still, there is an upside: Discovery of a concept gap gives you insight into your child's conceptual readiness for socialization, leaving you poised to work more effectively on the things that make socializing so difficult. And the process reveals what can be done to better accommodate, connect, and ultimately correct the misaligned frames of reference. We find a way over, under, around and through not only a child's concept gaps, but also our own.

Welcome to the Preparation part of The Connection Formula.

What Is a Concept Gap?

A concept gap is a fundamental difference in the way two people perceive how life works. When you perceive life in a unique way, your actions will probably appear quite illogical to anyone seeing things from the other side of the gap, especially if they don't know you are acting from a different viewpoint.

Is there a right and wrong side of the gap? It is best to sidestep that question for the moment, because such polarized thinking leads to another gap – the compassion gap – which I have mentioned earlier in the book. Let's start with the recognition that socializing is a two-way street. It involves mutual understanding in an agreed upon (yet unwritten) view of reality. All parties need the same frame of reference. This mutual frame of reference is often lacking between neurotypical and Autistic people, and this is the heart of the problem we have understanding each other. The missing frame of reference is what trips everybody up.

If few people think about the basic assumptions of the neurotypical social world, fewer still take the extra step to consider the rich alternative frames of reference unique to each child on the autism spectrum. We need to honor and respect those alternative viewpoints even as we try to explain our own.

* * *

In this chapter we will explore a wide range of concept gaps, representative of those you may uncover in your child's social understanding. Each gap you discover will jump up, wanting immediate correction. And it is our plan to address them. However, the matter of *when* and *how* is dictated by the nature of the gap, the emotional impact on your child, and the reliability of your communication. We want to motivate your child. We don't want them to feel beat up by the process. We don't want them to feel constantly *wrong*. We want them to feel connected. And so this part of the book is called *Connect Before Correct*. It's a reminder of priorities.

Remember, your child is probably not aware that there are any gaps in their understanding of life. Or they feel something is amiss, but misconstrue the nature of the gaps, so the concept of *concept gaps* itself needs to be introduced in a way they can understand and handle emotionally. And frankly, the same goes for you. Discovering these gaps is bound to have an emotional impact on any parent, so remember what I mentioned about the upside of these revelations. Each new discovery will give you a new way to gauge how difficult this all can be for your child, and will show you how best to help.

Also keep in mind that the problem of concept gaps is not entirely one-sided. Be on the alert for your own concept gaps in the examples that follow. There are many neurotypical blind spots, a topic I'll return to at the end of the chapter.

Imitation Without Understanding

Some people on the autism spectrum are able to copy those around them to a T. As a matter of survival, they become chameleons – actors who don't necessarily know they are acting. The better actors they become, the harder it is for others to figure out what's going on.

Donald was a brilliant scientist, but nobody could understand his written communication. Many simply assumed that his articles were over their heads; however, his inscrutable writing did receive criticism from some knowledgeable circles. What did he do about it? He tried to improve by copying a coworker. "People seem to understand your writing," he cheerfully informed his colleague, "so I'm going to use your topic headings." Sure enough, he had titled the different sections of his own article using headings from a recent paper written by the colleague. The trouble was that the borrowed headings had nothing whatsoever to do with Donald's content, which was now more inscrutable than ever.

Donald consciously imitated those around him in many other ways, with varying degrees of success. He had no feel for social conventions in the workplace, but managed to memorize the proper responses for most situations. With each misstep, he redoubled his efforts to imitate. He was brilliantly good at it, and even those who had caught on to what he was doing could still be fooled from time to time. That is, they were fooled into thinking Donald really understood the social conventions in the same way as everyone else.

How can you tell if there is real understanding behind someone's words and actions? Here's how: Watch for the thought patterns behind a conversation. They may follow unusual priorities and focus, weaving in different directions that at times make us mutually incomprehensible. Is there a shared intention, or does the conversation seem to be governed by unfamiliar rules?

A child with a gift for imitation may have no idea of the meaning of what they are imitating. Furthermore, they assume that everyone else is doing the same thing. They don't know they are doing things differently. This can be very subtle at times, and at other times it becomes strikingly obvious. I met one young man on the autism spectrum who repeatedly extended his hand in greeting throughout our conversation. Neurotypical conditioning made me feel rude when I resisted the impulse to shake his hand each time he presented it. Taking the pulse of the situation, I could see that he was completely unfazed. He had probably been taught to extend his hand when introduced to someone new, but had not been taught when to stop. Looking past his outer imitation of politeness, I saw a delightful fellow with a good heart who was happy to share a moment of connection, with or without a handshake. That is something to build on.

Unexpected Priorities

A child on the spectrum might assign unexpected weight to details that others barely notice. When an Autistic boy came into a treatment room and said, "Bonjour," his therapist was curious. She said to him:

👍 *Oh, you're talking French today. French is interesting. Is there a reason why you're speaking French?*

And he nodded yes, with a slight gesture toward a picture on the wall. It was a newly donated piece of art which he had never seen before, a painting of a seascape with a little ship in the distance, and on the ship was a flag no bigger than your fingernail. Can you guess the country? That's right: France. In the blink of an eye he had noticed the tiny French flag, and that's the detail he focused on.

Just as surprising is the information that a child might ignore.

A father told of the time he was driving his teenage son to meet Mom for lunch when they got a flat tire. Like most of us, the teen had often heard about the importance of being on time. On the other hand, he had never received instructions on the relative importance of fixing a flat tire. As bright as he was, this young man could not understand the need to stop and change the tire. In his eyes it was more important to be prompt. When this situation was brought to me, the father clearly did not think this sort of information needed to be taught; he believed his son should just automatically know about the dangers of driving on a flat tire and the damage it would cause. In fact, his son did understand all of that. Nonetheless, he assigned the flat tire a lower priority than being on time.

Some children with social learning disabilities will understand priorities on their own, and some will not. The misunderstanding in this situation wasn't at all surprising to me. There can be many concept gaps about priorities, so this is social information we will need to teach. (Chapter 15 offers a helpful approach for teaching about priorities that I call the "what's the bigger problem" game.)

Everything Can't Happen at Once

Thomas was an Autistic boy who would say, "Stop stealing my time," whenever there was a schedule to follow. Now this seems like a fairly normal reaction to a busy schedule, but Thomas means his words quite literally. He was not referring to his free time – he was speaking of time itself. I don't quite know how to explain it. Maybe this is the best way: Thomas thought that there would be time for everything if only people wouldn't put these limiting schedules in place. As we saw in Chapter 10, time is a slippery concept for some children on the spectrum.

We all know the frustration of not having enough time to do everything we'd like. For some Autistic children, this can be nearly impossible to grasp. For example, when it's time to leave the house for an appointment, you might give an early warning: *You can watch TV for five more minutes, and then we have to go.* It's not unusual for a neurotypical child to drag their feet in this situation, but a child like Thomas might be incapable of understanding why five minutes is not enough time to watch the remainder of a show. How can it be that departure time and TV schedules do not line up? There's a big difference between reluctance to turn off a TV and deep confusion when schedules play cruel tricks on your perception of time.

Perhaps some children simply can't grasp the concept of turning off a show before it's over, as if the length of the show itself is an indivisible unit of time, in conflict with other measurements such as hours and minutes, sooner and later, or the time it will take to drive somewhere. These things just don't match up in an easily explainable way. Time is not confusing to every Autistic child, but for some it is part of the chaos that surrounds them.

In a related area, distant memories can be just as vivid and have just as much impact as a recent one. I've mentioned before that the memory of an unsuccessful play date at a young age may still loom large in the emotional world of a teenager, it's painful impact undiminished by the intervening years. And yet at other times Autistic children have told me they feel fine about a recent traumatic event at school because, as we talk, they are safe in my office and the school situation is no threat in this moment. When back in school, the memory is more real and the threat is once again imminent. Time is indeed a slippery concept for some children on the autism spectrum.

Life Is Illogical

Life does not always conform to logic. Many of us no doubt wish it did. Some might not realize that it doesn't. How stressful life must be for those who miss this concept.

Have you ever been in a long line at the grocery store when a cashier opens a new register nearby? Often the last person in line just goes right over to the newly opened register and leaves the rest of us wondering, "Is that really fair?" Clear, rational thinking dictates that the next person in line should be given the right to go to the new register first. It's a perfectly logical way of looking at the situation, don't you agree? Of course life doesn't always work out that way. Common sense does not dictate how things actually happen, and rational thought does not always translate into the practical reality of day-to-day living. Neurotypical people tend to accept this. We may grunt in annoyance, but overall we take it in stride.

How does this work out from an Autistic point of view? Well, let me remind you that there is no one "Autistic" point of view, but I can tell you that I have had countless discussions with children on the autism spectrum who are surprised and confused by the illogical nature of life. A great many are completely disoriented when their perfectly logical thinking fails to change the world around them. Logic dictates their expectations, and when things don't work out in a logical way it can affect them deeply, causing frustration and confusion far beyond mere annoyance. It's hard for them to tolerate the broken logic.

Imagine that Laura, an Autistic teen, is asked by her mom to go hold a spot in line at the supermarket. Laura has in mind the "cattle gate" style of her favorite fast food restaurant, where everyone waits in a single queue for the next available cashier – a very logical system that achieves perfect fairness. This model of fairness is foremost in Laura's mind when she encounters the supermarket checkout lines. Where should she wait? There are too many lines! This could be profoundly upsetting to her.

Furthermore, repetition does not make the nature of neurotypical reality any clearer. This sort of concept gap usually does not sort itself out with more exposure to the situation. Every trip to the illogical supermarket continues to be illogical, out-of-balance, and frustrating. She's not going to suddenly unlearn the logic that makes it all feel so wrong. If Laura's social learning does not advance, it will never catch up with her logical processing.

To complicate matters, it is hard for someone like Laura to express what has gone wrong. Is she supposed to explain the source of her frustration to us? She might not even know that she is frustrated or confused. From her point of view, why would anyone need to explain things that are SO obviously illogical? To Laura and others who share this strong sense of logic it must look as if neurotypical people have lost their minds!

We adults have to be the confusion detectives and not leave it to the children to figure out the source of anxiety on their own. Yes, eventually we want them to be able to tell us what's going on – to find their own concept gaps, if that is even possible – or at least give us some description of what they think has gone awry. This is called *self-advocacy*. It's an advanced step that we are working up to. In the meantime, we have to be the ones to recognize and accommodate the concept gaps.

Disconnected Social Norms

We can all understand Laura's logic, and most of us would agree that people shouldn't get to jump ahead in line. But what if the child's logic is disconnected from social reality?

Tony learned in health class that if he is afraid of abuse at home, he can call a hotline and someone will protect him from the abusive relative. Tony does not live in an abusive home – he does not truly appreciate what this even means. But he doesn't know that he doesn't know, so he fits the information into the context of his own understanding and tucks away the pamphlet with the phone number.

One day Tony uses his dad's computer when he shouldn't. The computer crashes. Tony dreads the computer restrictions that will follow, so he calls the number and reports that he's afraid of his dad. The nice people will come and protect him. Small problem solved; big problem just beginning. I can assure you this sort of reasoning is not uncommon, though thankfully the consequences are not always so extreme.

Tony of course has no idea of the larger consequences of his "solution." It's not that he doesn't care about his dad or the trouble this will cause the whole family. He simply can't take in the full scope of what he has set in motion. His logic lives in isolation from the broader world, unencumbered by our social norms. Social learning and logical processing can be completely disconnected in this way.

Context Is Everything

For a child on the autism spectrum, an unseen inner logic provides context for their actions, their understanding of your questions, and the answers they give when you try to problem solve with them.

Brad always participated in class and worked on his assignments as expected – that is, right up until recess time approached. A half hour before recess, he stopped before his work was completed. Teacher and parents were concerned, and ascribed the behavior to his learning disabilities, then added on all the typical critiques: He was being lazy, irresponsible, not a "solid student." It was a daily problem, and as a consequence, every day he was held in from recess.

Of course I asked his parents if he liked going out for recess. The parents said, "Of course! Who doesn't like going out for recess?"

Well, I had my suspicions. Lots of children don't like recess. However, when I met with Brad I did not start with such a direct line of questioning. I did not want to go right to the heart of a potentially scary place. Even if he could face his feelings and translate them into words, he might not take the risk, as if expressing his truth would somehow be seen as a wrong answer in my eyes. *Context is everything.* His inner logic would likely miss my concern for his well-being, and instead make him feel like he was being forced to take a quiz.

On the other hand, he may well have replied that he liked recess just fine, since at that moment recess was not imminent. Asking a question about the past will often get you an answer that applies to now, not last week, not yesterday, not four hours ago. Again, *context is everything.* Brad might have no particular difficulty with recess while sitting in my office.

I also avoided the most direct and obvious question: "Why do you sometimes stop doing your class work?" Everybody else had already started with this question, and had gotten nowhere. Seldom will you get an accurate answer with such a broad approach. A child might not be a valid reporter of the reason – not because they don't want to answer correctly, but because they simply don't know how.

I advise parents against using direct inquiries. You *can* ask direct questions; just ask *safer* questions.

I started with smaller steps, leading Brad in a walkthrough of his day. I asked concrete, neutral questions. "Did you see Mrs. Smith? Was she wearing clothes you'd seen before, or new clothes? Did she say hi to you, or did she not say hi? Was your desk in the same place, or in a different place?"

Eventually we reached the key moment: "Oh, so you didn't go to recess because you didn't do your class work." Now of course I already had this information, but it was important to reach this moment of connection with him. When he confirmed with a subtle nod, I knew I was getting close.

"Was missing recess a problem?" I asked.

Brad replied, "Yes."

And I realized I had learned exactly nothing. Why? Because I had used the word *problem*. For Brad it was a poor choice of words. Yes, he had just told me that missing recess was a "problem," yet I could not assume that he meant missing recess was a problem *for him*. In other words, I still didn't know his feelings about it. The word *problem* has many connotations, and I did not know which meaning his inner logic had latched on to. To Brad, *problem* might not mean a feeling of displeasure, discomfort, or in this case the deprivation of a privilege (recess). There are other contexts in which the word is used. I know many children who enjoy doing math problems; for them the word might not have a negative connotation at all. Or perhaps my use of the word made no sense to him, and he simply gave a stock answer.

No harm done. If you find yourself at a dead-end or feel you have made a mistake with your words, just back up and ask a follow-up question. Even if you feel you understand a response, it's still good to cross-check the information you get in conversations like these; that's how you build reliable communication. So that's what I did.

"Did that bother you or did it not bother you?"

"It did not bother me."

Aha! From this point it did not take long to learn that Brad actually hated going out for recess, and would skip his class work precisely because the teacher kept him in from recess as a punishment. The behavior was not due to laziness, irresponsibility, or a learning disability, as everyone had assumed. It was in fact a well-planned coping strategy. He had solved the situation for himself, yet was unaware of the implications for everybody else.

There is plenty of confusion to go around. The adults misunderstand the child, and the child has no idea how the adults are seeing the situation. Some children are simply unable to come home and say "Recess is very hard for me." They don't know that this is an option, or they don't know how to explain the problem, or they don't even know that their negative feeling is a problem that can be explained and solved with the help of an adult. (This is a self-advocacy skill, which we hope the child will develop in time.) Adults suspect nothing until the problem manifests in some indirect fashion, as it did in this case. Then the temptation is to ascribe neurotypical reasons to the behavior. Child and adult are operating in completely different contexts.

What happens as a result? Well, think about Brad's case. What would have happened if we didn't get to the bottom of it? Do you think continuing the "punishment" would have helped? Can you keep upping the consequences?

You could make Brad miss every recess for the rest of his years in school and not be one step closer to the heart of the matter.

Where Are the Anchor Points?

Mathew was looking forward to a meal at McDonald's as a special treat at the end of a family outing, but it became a disaster before reaching the restaurant door. He had an emotional meltdown right there on the sidewalk for no apparent reason. What could have triggered this reaction? As it turned out, it was the wrong McDonald's. Not the usual neighborhood location, but a different location across town.

Even so, the meltdown was quite unexpected. McDonald's is McDonald's, right? How can Mathew be so fussy? Well remember Chapter 9. Change is a nightmare.

Some Autistic children seem to rely on familiar anchor points. When those anchor points are missing, a child can feel confused, disoriented, and even experience a sense of danger. To us, one fast food restaurant may be very much equivalent to another, but Mathew might have focused on some detail that we'd consider trivial, such as the curve of the walkway, a crack in the pavement, or the layout of the landscaping. Perhaps this led to the shock of realizing he was not where he thought he was, or the bigger shock of perceiving unexpected changes in geography. Or maybe he realized he wouldn't get his favorite booth or see familiar faces – more missing anchor points.

When you take such possibilities into account, suddenly a child's behavior is not so strange at all. If you saw life through their eyes, if experiences touched you in the same way, then you might very well react in the same way. Look through the lens of the behavior to the experience the child is having (not the experience *you* are having). To me an unusual behavior is a perfectly appropriate response to an unusual experience. We just don't know what that experience is like for the child. We think there's something wrong with the child's response. Instead, there's something missing from our own understanding.

Behavior for No Reason

How important is it to find the reason behind an unexplained behavior instead of dismissing it as part of the child's autism? See what you think in the following story that was shared with me many years ago. A parent reported that their seven year old Autistic boy had started hitting his nose and biting his hand "for no reason." When I hear the phrase *for no reason*, I immediately go on alert. Fortunately this child's therapist did the same. She did not brush it off as a behavior problem, and instead suggested that the child should be brought to a doctor. Care to guess what the doctor found? There was a bead in the child's nose.

Autistic children react to experiences we don't readily see, and they communicate to the best of their ability with whatever communication tools they have.

Neurotypical Blind Spots

I want to be clear about something (in case I haven't been clear already). When I refer to concepts that some Autistic people seem to be missing, this is not meant to imply that neurotypical people are in some way superior. I simply don't believe this is true. We can look at it another way, and ask why it is that neurotypical people take so many concepts for granted, especially concepts that don't hold up to the scrutiny of logic. I'm not asking you to question every ingrained convention of society, yet there are some concepts that we will do well to look at with new eyes. For example, many people (both Autistic and otherwise) do not understand the difference between social manners and social relatedness. Frankly, this is a huge blind spot that neurotypical people seem to have. We will explore the idea of social relatedness in Part 3 of the book, when we look at the importance of creating shared moments.

A related blind spot correlates intelligence with social awareness. Parents of children newly diagnosed with ASD have often said to me, "My child is so smart, how can they *not* be socially aware?" It somehow seems obvious to them that a high IQ automatically endows a child with good social skills. However, the two are not correlated, and if you assume they are it will lead to complications.

Intelligence and social awareness are not the same.

You need to recognize the difference. You tread on dangerous ground when you wrongly identify the motivation behind a child's behavior. Adults will claim, "He should know better," And in fifty other cases they might be right. However, an Autistic child does not fit the neurotypical profile. How unfair is it when a child is disciplined because an adult misunderstood? How much worse when that misunderstanding is due to the adult's own ignorance of the child's neurological makeup? These situations are incredibly harmful. Frankly, I've found that some school systems are slow to catch on to the difference between intelligence and social awareness, forcing families to prove the extent of their child's deficits, an awkward position for a parent if ever there was one.

Misidentifying the motivation for a child's behavior leads to an all-too-common scenario: easy victims grouped with bullies. Obviously this raises real concerns for the safety and well-being of Autistic children. It's not okay to be fooled by appearances when your decisions can put a child in harm's way.

Recently I've had the pleasure of working with a school system that fully embraces the idea of adjusting their frame of reference for each Autistic student. They are looking past the neurotypical blind spots, and it makes a huge difference in the progress they are able to achieve.

* * *

I am most interested in blind spots that impact the way Autistic people are treated. Here are a few unhelpful assumptions that neurotypical people make. (In case you don't notice, that's a "thumbs down" icon for each statement in **bold**. I am definitely not endorsing them!) I encounter these blind spots all the time, and I'll be touching on some of them again in the chapters ahead.

- 👎 **We all share the same frame of reference.**
  As you've seen in this chapter, basic assumptions about time, location, logic, priorities – and more – can vary widely. If you don't take this into account, there are lots of holes in the communication process. I call it Swiss cheese communication. If only the communication holes were as easy to see.

- 👎 **Repetition leads to learning.**
  Many use repetition to reinforce behavior, but do you know what behavior you're reinforcing? Without a mutual frame of reference, you do not. Perhaps you're reinforcing stress and anxiety: emo-

tional wounds to be healed. Or perhaps you're rewarding unwanted behavior so that Brad can avoid recess. Yes, a child will learn from repetition, but they will not necessarily learn what you're trying to teach.

👎 **If it seems rude, it must be rude.**
Neurotypical people are always misreading the intent behind an Autistic child's words. Remember what I said about Swiss cheese communication.

👎 **Eye contact will solve social problems.**
This is just one of countless variations on the mistaken idea that social manners have anything to do with social relatedness.

👎 **Autistic people don't have feelings.**
I hope I've already said enough to dispel this old myth.

👎 **Behavioral techniques can substitute for a mental health approach.**
Part of my work is healing wounds caused by simplistic application of behavioral techniques. A *significant* part of my work is healing wounds from a pervasive attitude about autism that allows this focus on behavior to thrive. That should tell you something about this particular blind spot. Look for compassion in the people who work with your child. Watch carefully to see if your child wants to follow their lead.

So you see, this is not a one-sided situation. It's not as if neurotypical people have some deep insight into autism that is simply not reciprocated. Frankly, the neurotypical view of autism is at times shockingly shallow. For better or worse, our neurotypical society holds all the cards. It is responsible for the social conventions and systems under which Autistic people must live, and it unwittingly impacts their well-being.

The important word here is *unwittingly*. This is a problem we can work on. I certainly hope there is no professional who would set out to emotionally harm an Autistic child, yet it is not rare at all to find children who have been harmed. I've tried to explain how this happens: it's those mixed up frames of reference that blind us to a child's concept gaps and prevent us from recognizing the real preparation that is needed.

Some say we cannot ever know exactly what is going on within an Autistic child's head. I have said as much myself, but we don't have to know *exactly*. We can know enough. How? By connecting with them in an authentic manner. An authentic connection let's a child show you how they think. True social relatedness is a miracle just waiting to happen, if you can clear the path. Each accommodation helps sweep away another obstacle. Each time you stretch your own conception of what life is like for your child, you strengthen the connection that is needed and more patterns emerge.

This is of the heart, not the head. Compassion combines with insight, love learns to speak through logic, and the greater goal of connecting with a child makes the outer social goals seem less important, while at the same time making them possible.

You and your child have much to learn from each other. When you can see their conceptual readiness for social information, you will know where to begin.

12

Emotional Readiness

Before we go too far into correcting concept gaps, we need to have some sensitivity about a child's emotional readiness for the process. We can't just start giving copious amounts of social information after we have uncovered a concept gap or two. How come? Why can't we just provide a one-on-one tutorial and teach all that is needed to bridge the gaps? Won't your child be happy to hear our information? Won't their quality of life improve quickly?

That would be nice, but it doesn't work out this way. A child needs to be emotionally ready to receive the information or our efforts will be wasted. Worse, we may set them back.

When I work with someone who is disoriented emotionally because of a concept gap, I start by validating their viewpoint. *Yes, you are right; this is confusing. It makes no sense.* Not only do we want to have reliable communication, we want to validate, validate, validate.

You may ask, *isn't this reinforcing an Autistic child's erroneous point of view?* No. It is *acknowledging* their point of view, and there is a big difference. I want children to feel good about who they are. I don't want them to be afraid of their own life. Can you imagine being afraid of day-to-day living? Life would be unbearable. That is not okay with me. First we connect and help a child feel safe in their own life. Slowly and steadily we earn their trust.

Having someone to trust is critical to a child's emotional well-being. We have to do all we can to be their trusted ally. They need to trust day-to-day life at home, at school, and in the community. I want to validate that the world *is* confusing, and I want to do this in a manner that does not create more anxiety. Our interactions with an Autistic child should feel like a relief to them. Adding more stress will not help you achieve your goal of a happier independent child.

Gradually, as a child is able to emotionally tolerate it, you can begin to delve more deeply into any conceptual gaps. First, though, we need to make sure the child can maintain their emotional equilibrium during this process. It may be uncomfortable for them at times, but overall the child should be feeling happier and happier.

You can start to see a rhythm to this, right?

Behaviors Reveal a Child's Emotional State

A parent wanted me to meet with school officials regarding their daughter's difficulty socializing with the other students. I'll call her Hazel. The school provided me with a log summarizing Hazel's day-to-day behaviors. Sure enough, it noted many ways in which she was socially isolated: eating lunch alone, not responding to questions, etc. – all things that the parent had mentioned to me. There were no real surprises…until I saw a note that the school was replacing the male aide with a woman who could find Hazel when she hid in the girl's room.

Wait – what? Hazel hid in the girl's room? This was a huge red flag related to her emotional state, yet it was barely a footnote in the daily log. This was the first thing I asked the school about. To my dismay, the staff didn't see how it was relevant. "It's just an autistic behavior," they told me. As it turned out, Hazel was spending ten or twenty minutes in hiding, several times a day, every day. This is a significant warning sign for anxiety, yet those who observed it dismissed it as just another peculiarity of autism. They didn't see that this was a child whose life at school was dominated by fear.

What amount of anxiety would cause *you* to literally run away and find a hiding place? Can you imagine this level of stress? Now imagine that those in charge seek you out and put you back onto the battlefield, where your survival seems to rely on arbitrary rules and unfamiliar concepts. I ask you, from the point of view of a child who lives in constant fear, could this environment be any less conducive to socialization? The school was defeating their own efforts because they did not see and acknowledge the fear in Hazel's life.

The school sincerely wanted to prepare Hazel for successful social interactions, yet whatever they were trying to teach, however they were trying to teach it, the lesson was completely lost on her. She was in no way emotionally prepared to receive the information or even recognize that any useful information was being presented. Quite the contrary, their approach left Hazel disoriented and confused. She was clearly struggling at a very deep level. I'm sorry to report that this particular school had little patience for discussions along these lines. To them, Hazel's "autistic behaviors" had nothing to do with her emotional state. Or perhaps they recognized the emotional underpinning of her behavior and simply dismissed it as unimportant. They apparently thought, as many do, that traditional techniques will work with Autistic children if we can just manage the behaviors, as if making behaviors go away will make autism go away. This would be very convenient for school systems, if only it worked. It most assuredly does not.

The situation is clearly very frustrating for schools (not to mention the frustration of parents). By and large, educational professionals have extensive experience and expertise for dealing with all sorts of behavior problems, and in this venue I am surely perceived as an outsider. I have had to face groups of passionate and dedicated educators and tell them that, in this one child's case, those tried and true techniques are probably going to fail. Truth be told, I am usually there because the techniques have already failed. However, I completely understand their skepticism toward trying something new. Learning about autism has been my lifelong passion. It is clearly not everyone's passion.

You can make it your passion.

Perhaps people steeped in traditional approaches find my way hard to accept because I do not wish to sweep aside the so-called "autistic behaviors." The behaviors are actually the key to making progress because behaviors reveal the child's inner world. Remember, for a confusion detective, behavior is the first clue to look at. It gives you a good idea of the child's emotional readiness. You cannot teach socialization to a child who is not emotionally prepared for it, so it behooves you to sensitize yourself to their emotional state. Behaviors are relevant. Please see them as valuable clues. When a child shows signs of anxiety, it is time to take a giant step back for some perspective. Fortunately, I have worked with some schools where such warning signs are taken seriously. There should be no controversy here; *all* schools should take this seriously.

To make progress with a child like Hazel, everyone must work to repair the damage that has been done and build a trusted relationship with her. Unfortunately Hazel's school was focused only on social skills. They were keen to make her socialize at all costs, so they pursued their agenda with single-minded purpose, steamrolling over this poor girl whose only recourse was to hide in the bathroom. I sincerely want to make everyone's life easier, but there is nothing I can do when adults are not willing to listen.

People want to change behaviors because they are the visible part of autism. I look at behaviors as a window into the child's world. I'm interested in reducing a child's fear, anxiety, and emotional pain. That must always come before addressing specific behaviors (as long as those behaviors are not dangerous to the child or others). You're not going to make autism go away by using behavioral interventions, so your goal should be to make a child's anxiety go away. This sets the stage for everything else you'd want for your child, and is why we must be able to evaluate and understand a child's emotional readiness for any change we wish to make and any help we wish to offer.

"Connect Before Correct" Moments

Jeremy was a four year old Autistic boy who barely spoke, so he had a preschool class assistant. During an activity, Jeremy said the word "book" for the very first time. This was an exciting moment for the assistant, who immediately went to fetch Jeremy's favorite book from a nearby shelf. That's when the teacher stepped in and said, "No, that's not what we're doing right now."

When did we become so rigid? That is a missed opportunity, and I find it very sad. We most definitely do things differently with The Connection Formula. To illustrate, here is a "connect before correct" moment from a socialization group:

Materials are stored in a red activities box in the treatment room. To keep things structured and focused, only the items involved in the

Emotional Readiness

current activity are removed from the box, which is positioned behind the therapist, out of the children's reach. Most of us would pick up on the social cue that the box is under the therapist's control and is not to be accessed by others in the group. Of course, social cues are difficult for Autistic children, so it was hardly a surprise when, at the end of an activity, one of the children ("Tumila") spontaneously jumped up and opened the box to take something.

This was a classic *connect before correct* moment. How did the therapist respond? Well, she did not scold. She did not say: *Tumila, sit down, don't touch the box.* She knew not to correct at that time. Instead, she simply observed: "Oh, you opened the red box!"

The therapist was well-trained in how to use simple facts to connect, using the approach described in Chapter 6. Here's how it worked out. Tumila responded, "I'm getting the next activity. All the activities are in here." And the therapist replied, "You're very smart – I like the way your brain works. Yes, that is where the activities are kept."

Do you see? So far this is all about connecting, not correcting.

Tumila did not know she was doing something wrong. Quite the contrary, she was very excited that she had figured out part of the system. It was a golden opportunity to connect. Correction (in this case, conveying the rules about the activities box) was far less important and could wait. If Tumila had been corrected immediately, would she have become upset? I don't know. Maybe. That's not the point. It's not a goal to avoid emotional reactions by letting children do anything they want.

The goal is to connect with them.

If that looks like coddling to you, if you feel this approach somehow produces an undisciplined child, then please take a closer look at what we're trying to accomplish. We do not avoid discipline; instead, we make it easier for all concerned. Connecting makes correcting easier, so we try never to miss an opportunity.

How are children going to learn if you don't correct them? Well, you *do* correct them. You need to choose the right time and the right way, as you'll see when we continue this example in the next chapter. In the meantime, consider this: are you teaching, or criticizing? Criticism has a cumulative negative effect. It is *not* a way to connect.

Aligning Your Frame of Reference

For every child on the spectrum with an undiscovered concept gap, there seems to be a neurotypical adult who misreads and misunderstands them. It is our job to *assume* there are concept gaps. And where there are gaps, there is inevitably miscommunication. So assume that, too. Miscommunication is not something that happens just once in a while. It happens frequently throughout the day.

If you're trying to teach an Autistic child to socialize, what do you do? Well, most people go with what they know about neurotypical children. For example, say Samantha comes into the classroom and always wants to sit in the blue chair. The teacher decides it's time to teach flexibility, and devises a plan to have her sit in a red chair instead. Perhaps the teacher simply removes the blue chair from the room. In comes Samantha. There is no blue chair. The result: a disruptive meltdown.

Many such scenarios have come to my attention over the years. Sometimes it's a chair, sometimes a book, sometimes a favorite gadget or toy. Perhaps you have witnessed such a scene yourself. Someone decides to deal with a child's "quirks" – their rigidity, their shyness, their mannerisms, their class participation or lack thereof – and soon the adult finds themselves out of their depth.

This is a sadly typical example of disconnected frames of reference. Does the teacher have any idea what's happening in the child's head? When I consult in school systems, I find that some teachers *think* they have a pretty good idea. And they would be absolutely right, *if* they were dealing with a neurotypical child. But when the child is Autistic, I have to ask this awkward question: are all the teacher's years of training and experience leading them to exactly the wrong approach?

If there's a wrong side of a concept gap, this is it: being unaware that the gap exists at all. It's time to back up and start with a different frame of reference.

Among other things, autism is a social learning disability, so let's use the social components of this scenario as our frame of reference. In our example, the teacher is not thinking of their blue chair intervention as a social interaction, but that's exactly what it is, and one that has very clearly hit this child where she is vulnerable. Think of Samantha walking into a room full of kids and not finding her usual chair – is that not a social interaction? The teacher interacting with Samantha about the situation – is that not a social interaction? Everyone watching and reacting as Samantha has a meltdown in front of the whole class – is that not a social interaction? Every interaction is a social interaction.

Autism impacts Samantha's social learning and her ability to perceive social expectations. We don't (yet) know the reason why she is so attached to that chair. Even so, can we really be surprised at a strong reaction when someone tampers with an Autistic child's frame of reference without understanding it? All too many would treat her meltdown as a behavior problem. But really, who created the problem here? Does anyone really think this child is "acting autistic" deliberately? I'm sorry to report that yes, many people tend to measure the complicated neurological challenge known as autism with the same yardstick used for neurotypical misbehavior, simply because that is the only frame of reference most people know. If autism were a culture, I would say that we are culturally unaware and insensitive. If autism were a language, it's as if we have no dictionary with which to translate.

What is the alternative? In a situation like this, I ask: What could be going on in this child's mind? The answer: I simply don't know.

But I can ask myself *what if*...

Think *What If*

What if, from Samantha's point of view, the world is so confusing that she tried to create a mental model to make sense of things? And *what if*, in this model, something about that favorite chair (or book or toy or gadget) is a constant she relies on: an anchor point. Perhaps it's simply the color blue. *What if* blue, in her world, brings comfort and helps her navigate daily living and all social interactions. Once you understand the reason for *blue*, or even attempt to find the reason for *blue*, then you've started to establish a mutual framework.

That is how I autism-ize my thinking.

As you consider the *what if* possibilities, how does that change the way you interact with a child? Do your priorities change? Do any new approaches come to mind? Even if your guesses are wrong, can you begin to see the need to tread more carefully? I find that thinking "what if" most definitely shifts my frame of reference, and that is one of its benefits.

Just as importantly, how does this approach change the way a child sees you? In our original scenario, Samantha comes into class to find a shocking change: her anchor point is missing, and the teacher has some stern lecture that makes no sense. Instead of removing the blue chair, what if the teacher had simply used a 1-5 safety scale to ask, "How do you feel when you sit in the blue chair? How do you feel if you have to sit in the red chair?" Do you see what a difference this can make to relieve a child's daily stress level? Someone is actually reaching out and offering a way to communicate.

A *what if* scenario is an educated guess. An "aha" moment may come all at once, or insights may creep in a little at a time. In the meantime, we are finding ways to connect with a child, and this lets them see us as an ally, a trusted social coach in the making.

Do we always guess right? Of course not. Yet when you guess enough – and test your guesses by using various accommodations and watching the child's reactions – then you will be led to priceless insights about the child's perspective. For me, a *what if* exercise always sparks new ideas for connecting to a child on the autism spectrum.

Know Your Impact

Imagine a first grader on the spectrum who is sent to the principal's office every day for being rude, disrespectful, and disruptive. Let's call him Elliot. Perhaps Elliot leaves his seat without permission and wanders around the classroom. He interrupts the teacher without raising his hand. One day he might jump up and erase something from the whiteboard in the middle of the teacher's lesson. Something like this happens every single day, multiple times a day, to the teacher's enormous frustration. Fed up, she sends him to the principal's office – again and again – yet the situation never improves.

Why?

Clearly Elliot has much to learn about how to behave in the classroom. Just as clearly, nobody has figured out how to teach it to him. Everyone is assuming they know the motivation behind his behavior, but they are not using the right frame of reference.

Some suggest that we need to reinforce the appropriate behaviors and discourage the less desirable behaviors. Yet when a child has autism, you cannot be sure what behavior you are really reinforcing. You think you know, but you may be quite wrong. Remember our story about Brad in the previous chapter, who wanted to skip recess and found a way to manage the behavior of adults who, ironically, thought they were managing him. He had worked the system to his advantage, as he perceived it. Far more often, Autistic children perceive a system set up to work against them.

Either way, typical consequences fail when they don't mean the same thing to an Autistic child as they do to a neurotypical child. The punishment does not fit the crime, so to speak, because in the child's view of the world no "crime" has been committed, and consequences therefore appear arbitrary and unfair. A reward may be seen as a punishment, a punishment as a reward. And a child will not relate either one to their own behavior if they are unable to objectively perceive their behaviors as you do. The conceptual differences leave a big gap between what you think you will impact and the actual effect you will have. Consider this: a child's emotional world may be so full of fear that they see everything they do as an act of self-preservation. If you don't grasp this world-view then you do not know your impact. Cause and effect is working, but can you be sure exactly what effect you are having? I think not.

Elliot is unable to learn expected classroom behavior by watching the other students. And he will not learn the rules through typical consequences because he does not perceive cause and effect the way you do. Let's all admit that continuous visits to the principal's office are not going to help him untangle the confusion of his school day. Whatever consequence you are applying, if it didn't work the first time or the second time or the third time, what makes anybody think it will work after the hundredth time? Perhaps Elliot actually likes the principal's office; maybe he feels safe there. In this case you are reinforcing the very behaviors you're trying to change, as we saw with Brad's strategy to avoid recess. Or maybe Elliot truly hates being in the principal's office, but can't understand how it relates to anything under his own control, in which case you are only adding to his confusion and anxiety.

The Connection Formula

The adults believe they see a connection between behavior and consequence. They do not understand the real reasons behind the behavior, so the connection they see is a false one. If the teacher does not make the connection and the principal does not make the connection, how do we expect the child to make the connection?

You need to make the connection.

Begin the Connection Process

So how do we deal with Elliot's behavior? You begin a process. For the moment, forget about correcting and try to imagine the situation from his point of view. You can begin to make a connection by considering some possibilities:

➢ **What *if*** his "wanderings" include a stop at the sharpener because he can't tolerate a dull pencil?

➢ **What *if*** the teacher had spelled a word wrong on the whiteboard, and Elliot was trying to be helpful by correcting it?

➢ **What *if*** he was enthusiastic about the subject matter and interrupted the teacher because he just wanted to participate?

These are all very real possibilities. (I encourage you to stop and think of some other plausible scenarios.) Would you agree that this casts a rather different light on Elliot's behavior? He might have no idea that he is seen as rude or disobedient. He might, in fact, have no idea what sort of behavior those words refer to. He is not deliberately breaking rules if he does not know those rules exist. He may even be trying to follow some rules quite literally: *Neatness counts,* so he keeps his pencil sharp. You get the idea.

The process continues by engaging Elliot without intimidating him. Remember, he needs to feel safe and understood. Here's how a teacher could use the running commentary technique from Chapter 6 in this kind of situation:

👍 *Elliot, you're out of your seat to sharpen your pencil so you can do your math work. I always like to see children who do their work...and you do need a pencil to do math!*

👍 *You're erasing the board. You must have a very good reason for doing that.*

👍 *You are very interested in technology and you have lots of information to share.*

Running commentary will not provide an instant solution. These are just opening statements, so to speak. But they are connecting statements, and they will put you on the right path. They get us away from neurotypical thinking, and they can actually help a child feel a bit safer. When connecting statements are the first thing to come to mind, you have made a very good start.

> **At Home and At School**
>
> I'm using a lot of school scenarios in this chapter because they show the emotional landscapes that Autistic children must navigate and the misunderstandings they continuously face. I hope you see that the principles also apply at home. Honestly, it has to begin at home. If you bring these ideas to your child's teachers, you might get more than one blank stare (I surely have). On the other hand, it's not out of line to ask what the school is doing to help your child feel safe and understood. Perhaps they will be part of a happy trend I've noticed in my local area, where more than one school is paying close attention to the emotional and conceptual readiness of their Autistic students, and learning creative ways to work with them.

Leading the Behavior

Eventually we would like to stop the behavior entirely. This is the result that everyone is rushing toward, but the rush to behavior modification is exactly what I'm asking you to avoid. We would like to correct the behavior, but correction does not refer to discipline. I use the word in the sense of correcting misunderstandings, bridging concept gaps, and providing social information (such as classroom rules) in a way that the child is well prepared to receive. If you do not have all of this in place, you are correcting in the dark. It simply doesn't work. You have to bring in the light.

Connecting brings in the light. Assume there are reasons for a child's behavior, then put on your detective hat and start looking for those reasons. Remember, no child is purposefully "acting autistic." It's not a behavior problem, it's a neurological difference. Correcting in the dark compounds the difficulty by creating confusion, anxiety, and all manner of related emotional problems. What you might see as autistic behavior is often the child's attempt to keep emotionally safe amid all this stress and confusion.

On the other hand, if a child feels safe, the defensive behavior is not needed. It's quite possible, then, that at least some of the concerning behaviors will improve. Connecting is not the whole story...but then again, it is. Everything starts with it. It gives you a way to lead the behavior.

Can Elliot's behavior be redirected without humiliating him in front of everyone? Let's say he left his seat to write something on the whiteboard. Understandably, the teacher might want to know what he's going to write before letting him share it with the whole class. For a child like this, the teacher might keep a small whiteboard on her desk. Here's one way to redirect him:

👍 *Oh, I see you are going to write something with the red marker. Can you write it on this small board first? I really want to see it. Then we will decide what to do.*

Notice how this starts with a connecting statement before leading the behavior in another direction.

This is labor-intensive in the beginning. You want everyone on the same page. Perhaps there is a paraprofessional in the class who uses the *connect before correct* principle. Hopefully Elliot's therapist will evaluate his emotional readiness and offer suggestions. In the perfect world, these suggestions are well received by the school staff. Ideally everyone is on the lookout for concept gaps, trying to discover the reasons behind the behavior. A team effort is required.

Always remember that you are trying to connect. Your tone of voice is not to discipline. If you are disciplining when you speak, you have to consciously shift away from that feeling. Yes, it's a challenge. It can be rather subtle, so I hope you catch the spirit of this approach. The flavor of your communication is as important as the words you say.

Reprogramming Your Responses

When traditional discipline does not meet with success, the thoughts in a teacher's head might be:

- 👎 This student needs to learn not to interrupt; he is disturbing the entire class!
- 👎 He is not an easy child to like.
- 👎 The consequences need to be stronger.
- 👎 He must enjoy getting attention from me, even though it is "negative" attention.
- 👎 I need the behavior specialist to create a very strict behavior plan for this.
- 👎 He is annoying and rude.
- 👎 He needs to learn how to respect authority.
- 👎 I'm going to repeat the same consequences until he finally gets it.
- 👎 This student is stubborn!

These are very common reactions, all perfectly understandable. Not one of them is helpful.

Because the child's concept gaps are invisible, the related behaviors are easy to misconstrue. This is a common experience for everyone, including me. I can honestly say that this is not easy to do. Reprogramming our responses is the key to discovering the missing concepts.

The Connection Formula

The first thoughts in our head need to be something like this:

👍 This situation needs further exploration.

👍 What concept gaps could be causing the behavior?

👍 Even though I feel disrespected, I can't assume the child intends it that way.

👍 I need to be patient to figure this out, even though patience does not feel natural in this situation.

👍 How is my student confused? I wonder what confusing thing happened that I totally missed.

👍 What rules were not explained in a way that makes sense to him?

👍 What miscommunication went unchecked?

👍 How can I see this from the child's point of view?

👍 I need to think *what if...what if...what if...*

That can be a lot of reprogramming! Let me break it down a little more by focusing on one type of situation that requires us to reprogram our responses.

I know both teachers and parents who have been offended by the words of children on the spectrum. A child may correct your facts, dismiss your suggestions, disparage your opinions, and even question your motives. This usually comes across as more than a little rude and disrespectful, and adults typically react according to that impression. It is painful to hear hurtful comments, especially coming from a child you are trying to help. Believe me, I understand the feeling. If a neurotypical person bluntly told you, "That is a really dumb idea," – or in a sharp tone of voice stated, "That movie you like is terrible!" – it would be off-putting to say the least. An Autistic child's comments can catch you even more off-guard, and feel like an overwhelming and exhausting barrage of logic and confrontation.

Here is how I handle it. First, although I try not to take it personally, I do allow myself to acknowledge the uncomfortable feeling.

Second, I imagine that if I feel hurt then the child may feel hurt, too. It's possible that the child has been hurt in the past, and I have simply stumbled into an area of sensitivity.

Third, I consider that the child's logical view of the world has been challenged. A trivial difference of opinion – even a misunderstood compliment – can put a child's internal logic process under stress. I always try to reinterpret the child's behavior, looking for alternate explanations that suggest a calm and helpful response.

The next step varies depending on my relationship with the child. If I am just getting to know them then I let the behavior slide for now. I need to develop and use accommodations, uncover conceptual differences, and assess the child's emotional readiness before I consider how to address the behavior. Also, I need to build trust, which is most definitely *not* nurtured by confrontation. Once trust has been established, there are times when I am able to directly let a child know how their behavior gets interpreted, providing useful social information in a gentle and factual way. For example:

👍 *When you say those things, some people might think you are being mean, but I know you are not a mean person.*

Don't be offended if someone on the spectrum corrects your facts or questions your motives. It is not necessarily meant as an insult. Don't assume you know the intent behind the behavior. Often the child is simply being honest, trying to keep their world in order. Or they may actually be trying to connect with you, even though their attempts come across as disrespectful and hurtful. Rudeness is a complex concept. We'll touch on it again in the next chapter. Your first step is to reprogram your response. Take it all in and let it show you how much help and compassion your child is going to need.

* * *

I hope this chapter helps sensitize you to your child's emotional readiness for socialization. Conceptual and emotional readiness go hand-in-hand in this journey.

13

Own the Misunderstanding

When a child on the autism spectrum does not understand a social convention in the neurotypical way, it is through no fault of their own. Therefore they should not be blamed for it or feel bad about it. No one wants to get corrected on a daily basis and continuously hear about all their social missteps. That's emotionally exhausting. This is especially true if you have no idea how to avoid the mistakes in the future. If we are unable to give social information in a way that a child can understand and assimilate, then that is *our* problem—not theirs.

A child in this situation may create some type of coping strategy as protection from this barrage of bad news. They might tune out, change the subject, have a meltdown, politely agree (even if they don't), apologize (not really knowing why), or isolate themselves.

There is a way to avoid all these bad options for your child:

➢ First take responsibility for the misunderstanding.

➢ Then provide the basic information that the child is missing.

Recall the story about the red activities box from the previous chapter. When Tumila opened the box without permission, the therapist responded with simple facts. (*You opened the red box. Yes, that is where the activities are kept.*) The therapist did not try to correct her in that moment. Now the time is right.

How will the therapist teach about the activities box? She will first make sure Tumila knows that she's not in trouble for missing the social cues:

The Connection Formula

👍 *Oh, I never told you who was in charge of the red box. That was my mistake.*

Always own the misunderstanding. Then go on to give information:

👍 *I am in charge of the red box. You can look at the schedule and tell me what to get for the next activity. You're very smart for knowing what's in the box.*

And that is the essence of this approach. I call it the *Did anyone ever tell you* technique.

Did Anyone Ever Tell You...

I find this approach particularly effective when trying to give helpful information without sounding like a know-it-all. The intent is to be apologetic on behalf of all adults who have been negligent by not giving the information in the past. You are the person who has come to the rescue, helping to free your child of embarrassment, criticism, and general emotional discomfort.

When your child makes a social misstep, tune your compassion meter to their point of view. Before you break down the social information related to the situation, you need to own the mistake that this information was never properly conveyed before. Begin by saying:

👍 *I'm sorry nobody told you...*

👍 *Adults were supposed to tell you...*

👍 *Did anyone ever tell you...*

There are many variations. The exact phrase is not important. Acknowledging and correcting the misunderstanding is. This is the whole "connect before correct" philosophy in one technique. It's very flexible and can apply to virtually any common (or unusual) concept gap, as the examples that follow will show.

Own the Misunderstanding

About Change and Surprises

A popular restaurant chain in the region recently closed a number of locations, including one just down the street from my office. A good many of my clients knew the restaurant well, and were understandably upset. It was very hard to conceive of the possibility that this anchor point could disappear, and the world seemed more than a little unstable to them when they learned the news. This was definitely a nexus of concept gap and emotion. How could I help them understand?

I used a very animated tone of voice, as if I just remembered something very important that nobody ever bothered to tell them. (And in fact, that was exactly the case.)

👍 *Did anyone ever tell you that restaurants do not stay forever? Some restaurants are there for a long time, but that does not mean they will always be there. Some restaurants are owned by big companies, and some are owned by just one person. This restaurant is owned by a big company and still has other locations, so you might have your favorite meal again.*

My favorite Italian restaurant is owned by a married couple. When they retire, they will probably close the restaurant and I will have to find another favorite meal. New restaurants open, too. It will be exciting to see which new restaurants open on the roads where you and your parents travel.

The closed restaurant is an example of a "bad surprise." When we get to problem solving (Chapter 16) I'll suggest ways of creating a bad surprise plan. Before we get there, you may find it necessary to teach about surprises both good and bad:

👍 *There are changes that you might expect, like school beginning in the fall. Changes that we don't expect are called surprises. Some surprises are good, like getting a gift from your parents when you didn't know they were going to buy it. Some are bad surprises, like going to a movie that you really want to see but there are no more tickets left. We cannot always control changes and surprises.*

About Idioms

When the teacher says, "Take your seat," what happens if a child literally moves the chair to another part of the room? (Yes, this really happens.) The teacher is frustrated. The child is confused. We can accommodate by avoiding idioms, but how do we work toward correcting the problem?

First you need to consider your child's emotional readiness to bridge this misunderstanding. Are they ready for direct feedback? Don't assume so. You can begin by throwing out a lifeline.

👍 *That is a very logical way to understand 'take a seat.' I like the way your mind works.*

Next, to teach the meaning of the idiom, you should own the misunderstanding:

👍 *Did anyone ever tell you about the 'take your seat' expression? I'm sorry that I never explained it. When the teacher says to 'take your seat' they do not mean to take it away. They mean for you to sit in your seat.*

I always like to normalize the mistake so that the explanation does not sound punitive.

👍 *Did you know you're not the first one to think that? Yes, it is confusing. The expression is not logical. It is hard to understand when people don't say what they mean.*

Every child is different, and every parent brings their own style to this technique. The process can take time. Will your child immediately be able to generalize what they learn about one confusing idiom and extend it into all confusing areas of life? No, this is usually not a realistic expectation. However, one thing that does generalize to other areas is your child's trust in you as a source for social information that makes their life easier. Trust makes it possible to move things forward a little at a time.

Own the Misunderstanding

About Fairness

I often play simple children's games in socialization groups. The games are a microcosm for things a child will experience in the wider world, where life does not always seem fair. How well prepared is a child for socializing outside a therapeutic environment if they have a meltdown when they don't get a match in a card game like Go Fish?

I help prepare them by presenting social information in a very matter-of-fact way.

👍 *Didn't anyone ever tell you life is not always 100% fair? Some things do not seem fair, like when other players have more matches in Go Fish than you do. Other things are really not fair, like being blamed for something you didn't do and getting sent to the principal's office because of it. The card game uses luck, and luck cannot be fixed. But we can try to fix the things that are really not fair.*

It is important to have more fair things than not fair things in life, but we can't always fix everything.

About Compliments

A child once said to me in a group "Every week you tell me that you like me. Do you think I'm stupid?" A lot of adults would think the child is being disrespectful, even belligerent. In reality, the child actually thought that I was repeating myself because I thought she didn't understand me. My weekly compliment was hurtful to her! I owed her an explanation:

👍 *Did anyone ever tell you about compliments? Often people repeat them because they think you'll like hearing positive things again and again. It's not because they think you're dumb and forgot that you heard it before. People like giving compliments because it shows they like you and they think you'll enjoy it because it's like getting your favorite dessert again and again.*

Here's another way to explain compliments:

👍 *Didn't I ever tell you? When I think about you, I think many positive and good thoughts. I like these thoughts because it makes me happy. Saying a positive thought out loud is a compliment. Then you know I am thinking good thoughts about you. I give you compliments because I think they will make you happy, too.*

About Rudeness

Years ago one of my nephews asked his grandmother if she had a hot date. (Granny had gotten her hair done and had a new outfit; she was looking pretty good!) We all laughed. It was fun and good-natured. Now can you imagine if my nephew went to school and asked his principal this same question? It would probably be considered rude and disrespectful. Politeness and manners can be very confusing. A child cannot talk with a teacher the same way they can talk to a beloved family member.

👍 *Did anyone ever tell you that being rude usually means you have done something that is not nice? There are many different types of rudeness and it can be very confusing.*

Most adults do not explain all the different types of rudeness. It is an adult's responsibility to teach children about rudeness so they don't get in trouble.

Some very well-meaning parents believe that having autism is no excuse for being rude. That is a view of autism through neurotypical glasses. I agree that social manners and being polite are important; you just have to teach it differently. Make sure you include information about *why* something is considered rude.

It helps to look at three different categories of rudeness. The first concerns social manners like saying *please* and *thank you*. An Autistic child may neglect to do these things due to lack of awareness. There is no desire to be impolite; it is literally a missing concept.

👍 *Did anyone ever tell you why people use manners like* please *and* thank you? *Manners let people know that you are trying to be nice.*

Own the Misunderstanding

The second category of rudeness concerns more personal interactions. Everything from daily conversations to arguments and conflicts are in this category. Again, there are social norms in place that children on the autism spectrum might be unaware of. For example, some children might not know they need to answer when someone asks a question. For such a child there may be no emotional weight to staying silent, although neurotypical people usually interpret their silence as rudeness. Other Autistic children don't answer because of anxiety, a different situation entirely, but it appears just as rude to the person being ignored.

👍 *Did anyone ever tell you that people might think you are rude if you don't answer them? They might think you are being mean to them and don't like them. If you don't know what to say, then 'I don't know' is an okay answer.*

The third category is when a child is annoyed and does not know an appropriate way to express it. A child might not even realize that people can see they are annoyed or hear it in their voice. They haven't learned to self-observe.

👍 *Did you know that people can see when you are annoyed even if you don't tell them? That's why it's important to know how you're feeling when you're talking to someone.*

Use this technique judiciously in order to maximize its positive impact. Don't use it as a veiled way to modify behavior. Do NOT say: *Didn't anyone ever tell you to say please and thank you? Did anyone ever tell you that you're rude?*

Do not correct the child. Correct the *misunderstanding*.

When a child acts in a manner considered to be rude, adults will usually take it as a sign of disrespect. Respect is a very difficult concept to explain. You might do best to say it means not being rude, and build the concept from there.

Certain Autistic children are somewhat aware of the concept of respect. Often they need to be shown – gently and over time – just what it means and how to gauge the respectfulness of their words and attitude. It's a very subtle area. Some children are surprised to learn how their words and demeanor are perceived by others, and don't understand why it gets them in trouble. I want them to know the reasons behind the cause and effect. Trust me, you cannot do much along these lines until you establish reliable communication. That's why we put accommodations in place before jumping head first into deeper waters.

About Mistakes

Does your child understand that people have different strengths and weaknesses? Do they know that people don't have to be perfect? In arithmetic, 2+2 is always 4. There is no room for any other answer. As you know (although a child on the spectrum might not), people aren't like number problems. Thinking in black and white terms about human relationships leaves out most of the picture; so does thinking about oneself in absolute terms. For example, not getting a score of 100 on a test could be devastating to some children.

👍 *Did anyone ever tell you? Everybody makes mistakes. That's why they have strikes in baseball. Do you know how many times a baseball player might strike out before they even make it to the major leagues? Too many for me to count! That does not mean they are bad baseball players. All baseballs players strike out sometimes. All of them! 100%!*

In some of my socialization groups, when I feel group members need help with this concept, I will keep track of my own mistakes. I count everything from interrupting someone to forgetting the art supplies in another room. Trust me; the number of little mistakes one makes in 45 minutes of interactions is surprising. Incorrect grammar, calling a child by the wrong name, dropping something on the floor...it's not hard for me to find examples. Believe it or not, in order to demonstrate that it's okay to not be perfect, I encourage the children to point out all of my mistakes. Yes, I have to be thick-skinned about it! I do this because it shows them that everyone does make mistakes. I'm giving them data in a way that is fun for them. You see, it's not enough to tell them that making mistakes is okay. You have to prove it. As they tally my errors, I say, "I'm not a bad person when I make mistakes. I don't feel badly when I make mistakes, and you can still like me when I make mistakes!"

> **Free Pass Cards**
>
> When a child has difficulty tolerating their own mistakes, I sometimes recommend giving them some "free pass" cards. When they make a mistake they can use a card to get a "free pass" and make it all okay. Of course even without the card it is all okay. (You weren't going to punish the child for an honest mistake, right?) The cards are mainly to help with the child's anxiety, to relieve them of the need to be perfect. The cards are tangible proof that perfection is not necessary. Otherwise the child is faced with the prospect of somehow being a "wrong human being," a truly distressing thought for them.
>
> There is another benefit: When your child uses a card, it helps make their emotional world visible. You learn what they view as mistakes, and glimpse how this makes them feel.
>
> Free pass cards work at home or at school (as long as the teacher is in on the plan). For example, a child might turn to the wrong page in a school book. On realizing this, they can give the teacher a mistake card, "I made a mistake, I read the wrong page." The teacher makes it okay to have made the mistake. "Everybody makes mistakes. You did a good job finding it!"

About Logic

Jayden strongly objects to homework, but his objections are not based on lack of interest or discipline. He enjoys most subjects at school, yet for him homework is truly illogical. For example, he does not feel he needs to do twenty of the exact same type of math problem in a row. He thinks it's stupid, and would rather learn something new. Why is someone else controlling my time (he wonders), especially when he already knows the material? His objections are so strong that he has considered writing to the State Department of Education about the illogical nature of homework. He believes they will immediately reform the system once he makes his point. His father talks to him about this:

> 👍 *Did anyone ever tell you that logic does not change reality? Logic is important, but it is not always what makes things happen in life. Humans make illogical things happen all the time (like homework), and they don't even know it. Just because something is logical does not mean it is going to happen.*

Dad goes on to validate Jayden's viewpoint that homework is not always logical, then explains that logic does not change the reality that the homework must be done.

Taylor is going to help her mother make a cake. Her mother begins to fetch the ingredients as Taylor reads them from the recipe. Mom brings out the milk and eggs together, but milk is the last ingredient in the recipe. This upsets Taylor. "Mom, you're supposed to get the sugar next!" Mom recognizes the disconnected logic. Taylor has a logical way of looking at the order of ingredients in the recipe. To us her way appears rigid and literal; to Taylor the logic keeps the world in order.

Mom could accommodate her daughter's logic and do it Taylor's way to avoid a meltdown. That would be a good choice in the early stages of The Connection Formula. Instead, she makes a judgment call. This mom has many accommodations in place for communicating with her daughter (the problem scales are never far away), so lately she feels more confident about their interactions. Here's what Mom explains about logic as she puts the milk and eggs on the counter:

> 👍 *Did anyone ever tell you that people do not always use the same logic? My logic is to get everything I need from the refrigerator at the same time, so I will get the eggs and the milk together. Your logic is to use the recipe order. That is very good logic, too. But the recipe does not know how our kitchen is organized, so I am using different logic. We are going to mix a cake, and we are going to mix our logic!*

Here is a more general explanation of logic. Notice how we always start by validating before giving additional information.

Own the Misunderstanding

👍 *Oh, I see how your brain works; that makes sense; that is very logical. My brain works differently; these are my thoughts. It's okay that our brains work differently; do you agree or disagree?*

Not every child will find it easy to accept an alternate logic. There is another way to approach the topic when a child is upset by an illogical situation:

👍 *Did anyone ever tell you that people are not always logical? People who are illogical are not necessarily trying to hurt your feelings or be strange. They do not know they are being illogical. It is hard for their brains to think logically. They do not know they are confusing.*

An even more basic concept about logic can be explained this way:

👍 *Didn't anyone ever tell you that people do not all have the same thoughts in their heads? When you talk I can tell you have very good logic, but I don't know what logic is in your head unless you tell me.*

I encourage you to combine accommodations. Don't forget about the 1-5 logic scale. When you approach it in a light way, it can be fun to compare your differences in logic. If it is stressful for your child, don't force the conversation. Let them show you their view without trying to correct them. Always validate. "You have a very logical way of thinking." Then bring it forward from there. "Your teacher uses different logic..."

A Measure of Safety

Children on the spectrum are expected to take in lots of new social information on a daily basis. For us this may come easy; for an Autistic child, this might be akin to memorizing an encyclopedia. (Remember those? These days I suppose you could say we are asking them to memorize Wikipedia.)

The social learning process can feel punitive for someone with a social learning disability. Constant criticism and correction leads to low self-esteem and stress. When someone is stressed, it makes it even harder to take in new information. A child may become defensive and guarded. That is just one reason why counselors try very hard to connect with their clients before digging more deeply into emotionally charged issues.

When I work with Autistic children, I have to assume there have been some deep misunderstandings in their lives, on a level that can produce symptoms of trauma and loss. This often turns out to be the case, and I need to help heal that. I will apologize for a loss that has happened in a child's past. I have actually written letters of apology to children on behalf of institutions that have unwittingly failed them, and my apologies are always heartfelt and sincere. This validates the child's viewpoint and lets them feel a measure of safety as we build more trust.

Own the misunderstandings. Sincerely. I hope you recognize that phrases like *did anyone ever tell you* should never be used with a hint of impatience or sarcasm. If we've done a poor job of connecting with children on the autism spectrum and teaching them our (sometimes illogical) ways, then let's own the problem and begin to do something about it.

14

A Concept Gap Journey

In the following case history I'll try to give you some idea of what it can be like to uncover and correct a concept gap while accounting for a child's emotional readiness. This process took place over many months. You simply can't push too hard when a child's emotional well-being is at stake.

"Luke" was in trouble at school for running out of the classroom every time a particular boy talked to him. The pattern seemed to be clear: Whenever this other boy approached him, Luke left the room. However, when teachers and parents asked Luke if he liked the other boy, he always said, "Yes." When asked if he had a conflict with the other boy, he said, "No."

This was an ongoing mystery for me as well, but it was a mystery I was willing to place on the back burner. I'd been meeting Luke regularly for just a short period of time, and my priority was to build a connection, working with various accommodations to establish good communication. If I simply repeated the same questions already asked by parents and teachers, I was not likely to get any new information. If I don't have my accommodations in place, then trust has not been established and communication is not reliable.

When I began to work with Luke I was – as always – on the lookout for concept gaps, hoping to spot any difference in his awareness of the unspoken, mutually agreed-upon way in which neurotypical people look at life. Don't confuse this with how one *acts* in life. Actions – behaviors, the quirks everyone is always trying to "fix"– arise from how somebody perceives the world and how they think of themselves in it. Behavior is the visible surface of something much deeper. It is in

The Connection Formula

the deeper area that the concept gaps are found.

Was there a concept gap behind Luke's behavior? Almost certainly there was, although it's not something you can easily ask about. Yes, there are ways to try. Using our best literal language, we can try something like this:

> 👍 *You are getting in trouble. You seem to be a very nice boy. I know you have good reasons for what you do. I would like to know those reasons.*

This is the kind of thing I have tried in some cases. It might work. Maybe. I don't do it often. Why? First, because asking some children directly about their behavior can be very scary for them; there will often be some emotional sensitivity involved. Second, if there is a big concept gap, the entire conversation might be meaningless and terribly confusing to them, and trust can be lost. So you have to consider their emotional and conceptual readiness in tandem. In Luke's case I proceeded carefully, and kept my eyes and ears open.

One day, after one of our sessions, I overheard the following conversation as Luke and his mom prepared to leave.

"We're not having carrots for dinner, are we?" Luke asked.

"No," said his mom. "I know you don't like them."

Luke's reaction was unexpected: "Mom, be quiet!" he snapped.

It was an unusual reaction; a possible clue. How could it relate to the issue with the other boy at school? I had no idea, so I tucked the information away for future reference.

On Luke's next visit I uncovered another clue. We were reading a book in which the main character makes a mistake. On reaching that part of the story, Luke made this comment: "I never do anything inappropriate!" It was another strong and unusual response, exactly the kind of thing you should be watching for. In particular, it was an odd use of the word *inappropriate*. What was "inappropriate" in Luke's world? I wondered, and decided it was time to put my clues together. While "playing" the *true or false* game (Chapter 6), I slipped in the following question:

> 👍 *True or false: Is it inappropriate to dislike carrots?*

Luke hesitated. Finally he said *true*, it was inappropriate. Here was the tip of the iceberg. A concept gap was about to surface, and I had no idea how far-reaching it would be.

> **Through a Child's Eyes**
>
> I am always pleasantly surprised when I discover the right question to ask a child. I know a concept gap is there, but I never know when or how it is going to reveal itself. When the moment comes, it feels like I've struck gold. Suddenly I have a view through a child's eyes. The whole story seldom emerges all at once, but at last I have what feels like a magic pair of glasses that lets me glimpse their world.
>
> It is always an exciting moment.

Sitting with Luke, there was suddenly a shape to my mission. I needed to learn why disliking carrots was "inappropriate," and figure out how such an idea could have sprung from the tapestry of his life. I felt a great anticipation. What else was I about to learn?

The first thing I needed to clarify for myself was in the area of language. What did Luke mean by the word *inappropriate*? The second area was more important: what did he label as inappropriate, and how did this color his experiences?

Working carefully over a number of sessions, I explored both areas using variations of the 1-5 problem scale and concrete questions about likes and dislikes. I made up scales in the moment, drawing them on a whiteboard. I used hand gestures and exaggerated expressions to represent the size problems. I took my time, and backed off of the topic whenever he seemed uncomfortable. We spent a lot of time simply connecting on unrelated matters that he was more comfortable with.

Over time I learned that in Luke's world, inappropriateness corresponded to a big problem (level five on my problem scale), and that pretty much anything that Luke disliked ranked as a level five on an "inappropriate scale." In other words, he thought that disliking a movie, a TV show, or a video game was inappropriate. He thought that disagreeing with people in any way was inappropriate. He thought that saying he was sad, angry, or confused was inappropriate.

For Luke, *any* negative feeling was inappropriate, and feeling inappropriate was no small thing. It meant "I am bad." As a result, he constantly tried to banish all such thoughts and feelings.

Of course Luke was unable to manage this. Who could? He thought that only bad people had thoughts about their likes and dislikes. Only bad people felt sad or upset. He wanted to be a good person. Can you imagine the daily stress he was under? His goal was literally impossible. Here was the concept gap, and it was a big one.

Still, there was more to come.

As I worked with Luke, the deep source of his anxiety became even clearer: he thought he was the only one in the world with likes and dislikes. He did not realize that *everyone* has these so-called "inappropriate" thoughts and feelings. We call them preferences, opinions, matters of taste and style. Nobody ever told him this was normal. In his mind he was alone, an outcast for preferring peas to carrots. And he believed that if he expressed his preferences, it would make matters much worse. He thought that expressing his opinions would somehow conjure negativity into reality, putting it out there for all to see. The world would know he was different, a bad boy, and that is the last thing he wanted to happen.

As Luke's view of himself sank into my awareness, I was very glad I had not pressed him too directly. I would have been charging blindly into his deepest fears about being a bad person – a child unworthy of love. I felt tremendous relief that I hadn't injured him. I felt privileged to witness what was really going on, and grateful that I hadn't jumped to conclusions about his behavior.

Also, I felt a burden. How was I going to convince anyone else that this was how he saw the world? It is for boys and girls like Luke that I wrote this book. And I wrote this book for you, so you would know why it's so important to autism-ize your thinking, and what it means to a child in need of a lifeline.

* * *

Before I conclude Luke's story, stop and consider how this hard-won awareness of his viewpoint changes your perception of him. I've shared this particular moment as one of many from my work in order to give you an appreciation of the delicate touch and degree of compassion required to help children like him. There is a definite

A Concept Gap Journey

philosophy behind The Connection Formula. I describe it with phrases like *safe and understood, connect before correct, get to know your child's world*. This story shows how that looks in action.

On a practical level, I hope to give you some ideas on how to proceed with behavior problems. Think about how many unusual behaviors might spring from Luke's unique view of the world. More than a few, for certain. A single *Eureka* moment can lead to an enormous amount of information to work with. When all of this information comes to light, the temptation is to race ahead. Now, though, is the time to once again slow down. Please be sure you have a grasp of your child's emotional readiness, and proceed accordingly. A single insight – even a big one – does not always bring an instant answer. It certainly didn't in Luke's case. What we look for is a starting point. We first need to know all the missing concepts, or as many as we can indentify. Then we need to work with the child's emotional readiness to communicate about the situation so they can eventually learn a happier way. My journey with Luke was just beginning.

* * *

The concept gaps here are plentiful. Luke was not consciously aware that he was hiding his feelings; he was just trying to do the right thing, to be a good boy. Here are some of the concepts he was missing; you may be able to think of more possibilities.

➢ Everyone has negative feelings.

➢ Not everyone likes the same things.

➢ People are allowed to have different opinions.

➢ Opinions are not facts.

➢ It is okay to have strong feelings.

➢ Expressing your feelings does not make you a bad person.

These are some rather important concepts we have identified. Now what? How do we know what Luke really feels about *anything*? How can a discussion about these concepts even begin? It seemed to me that Luke had a hard time tolerating his own thoughts and feelings – not because they were "bad," but because he *thought* they were bad. The last thing he wanted to do was discuss them.

My first goal was to increase Luke's tolerance for the subject of *differences*. Not his personal differences with others – he was not emotionally ready for that. So I focused on the idea of differences in general. I started with favorite things, such as favorite animals, colors, TV shows, etc. I did it very casually, in a matter-of-fact way. I explained that people have different favorite things, and owned the mistake that nobody had ever explained this before.

I then moved the topic forward from different things that people like to things that people *dislike*, a more highly charged concept. I talked about people disliking certain foods and how people's taste buds can physically differ, making them sensitive to different flavors. I used as many facts as I could to show the logic of this information. Disagreements over things we strongly dislike can be more pronounced, which Luke would have seen as inappropriate (i.e. *bad*). So based on Luke's responses I gauged how much information I could give, and how quickly. When he seemed stressed I slowed down the process.

After a few months of counseling, Luke was able to tolerate discussions of likes and dislikes. He was even able to openly disagree with me. (I happen to like carrots.) Yes, it was a long process, but we made big progress.

* * *

Now you're probably wondering about that situation at school. Why was it that Luke ran out of the classroom every time that particular student spoke to him? This was the situation that had brought him to me in the first place, and I had not forgotten about it. As you have seen, there were greater matters to deal with. In the rush to solve a behavior problem, it can be easy to miss the much more important hidden problems at the root of the situation.

At last Luke was conceptually and emotionally ready to discuss it. Here is what I learned:

Luke had lost several Uno card games to the other student, and felt badly about losing the games. As we now know, in Luke's world such feelings were not appropriate. He couldn't tolerate them, and did his best to keep them at bay. However, when this boy talked to him, Luke's memory of losing the games flooded back in, the associated negative feelings arose, and Luke felt very anxious and guilty – or, using his word, *inappropriate*. He needed to get away from the boy, and so he solved the problem by fleeing the classroom.

I hope you can appreciate that Luke's behavior was completely rational and logical – according to the rules of Luke's world. Since Luke believed that it was inappropriate to discuss the card games and his feelings about them, he had done a superb job of avoiding the topic. In Luke's mind he had solved the immediate problem of being a bad person by avoiding interactions with the other boy. Of course, leaving the classroom created new problems. This led to anxiety for which Luke had no ready solution. He was not even aware that he was feeling anxiety. In his words, he identified it as feeling *inappropriate*. He was certainly stuck between a rock and a hard place.

Now he is less stressed, and is a much happier child.

I hope this story shows you how deep some behaviors go. The internal logic of autism is always at work, and a child's well-being depends on our ability to uncover it.

15

Unconfusing the Rules

There are two sides to the issue of rules. On the one hand, rules help make social expectations clear in a confusing world; a child may focus on rules for consistency, safety, and comfort. On the other hand, rules can be intimidating, and some children feel the need to follow every rule to the letter. Perhaps this is because of their literal viewpoint; perhaps it is due to the feeling of safety that rules bring; perhaps it is out of a desire to be "good." No matter the reason, rules can create a great deal of anxiety because it is simply impossible for a child to follow all of the rules all of the time. Rules are confusing, easily misunderstood, and sometimes the means to obey them is beyond a child's control.

Imagine that the school bus makes Alan late for school. Obviously the delayed bus makes all the other kids late, too, but Alan's logic is focused on the perception that he has broken a rule about being punctual, and now he believes he will suffer the consequences. He may realize that nobody will punish him for the bus delay; nonetheless, walking late into a classroom can feel like a very big consequence. The bigness of the problem for Alan is out of proportion to our norms. He anticipates a very scary social interaction, and is so stressed by the situation that he unwittingly creates an even bigger problem: a meltdown on the bus.

It is not unusual for a child's desire to be "good" to lead them into "bad" behavior. Such is the level of anxiety that rules create.

Alan may come to understand it is not his own fault, but now that someone else (the tardy bus driver) appears to have broken a rule, Alan's sense of fairness and consistency feels violated, and the world seems unsafe and impossible to control. His logic dictates that the bus driver should be fired and arrested for causing this huge problem. The out-of-proportion bigness of the rule violation remains in sight and is seeking balance.

It should hardly come as a surprise that this varies greatly from child to child. If you begin to dig into the rule-following habits of Autistic children, you will discover that they do not all have the same level of understanding, nor do they all focus on the same rules. A rule-driven child typically has preferred rules – rules they rely on more heavily than others. Look at which rules your child ignores versus the rules they feel must be followed. Is it upsetting to your child when a rule is broken, either by themselves or someone else? Does your child understand if and when it is appropriate to be flexible about some rules? Just as importantly, do *you* understand why certain rules are important to your child?

The Tangle of Exceptions

Neurotypical people seem to have an innate flexibility about rules. As the expression suggests, we generally know the difference between *the letter of the law* and *the spirit of the law*. If your child is missing this concept, then even simple social rules can become an impossibly complex tangle of exceptions. Let's look at one example: the social rule about not interrupting others when they are speaking.

We learn as young children not to interrupt, yet in reality people interrupt each other all the time. If you don't believe me, just listen to neurotypical people who are engrossed in conversation. When people are excited about a topic they freely interrupt with related comments or clever quips as these come to mind. Often several people start talking at once. Sometimes it is hard to get a word in edgewise! This might not be a good model for a formal meeting, but it's certainly the norm in social gatherings and many everyday situations.

Here's another scenario where the rule doesn't apply. Say you are having a conversation at a restaurant. What happens when the server comes to your table? The server is expected to interrupt, and usually the conversation is put on hold while everyone places their order. So in reality the strict rule of never interrupting just doesn't hold up under scrutiny. Obviously some flexibility is needed.

Now let's imagine the impact of the "no interrupting rule" on an Autistic child. We understand that it has many exceptions. Does your child know them all? Does anybody? No one is going to make a complete list of specific exceptions because new scenarios come up all the time. The list would never end! We're all left to figure it out in the moment. The rule just can't be pinned down in a literal way, so where does that leave someone who relies on literal thinking? Can your child figure out when it is okay to interrupt and when it is considered rude? If you don't have a feel for social situations, it is impossibly complicated. Some children will figure out a few of the exceptions while missing many others.

Again, this varies from child to child. I have worked with children who feel absolutely horrible when they interrupt, when in fact they have done nothing wrong. A lively and fun discussion is taking place in a socialization group, and suddenly one of the participants freezes with a look of fear. I notice and immediately ask what's wrong. Too many times to count I have heard the following sort of response: "I interrupted, I'll stop talking now." And the child begins to shut down. In reality they never actually interrupted in a manner that might be considered rude. They were adding to the conversation in an eager and socially acceptable way, yet they could not enjoy the social experience because they thought they had broken a rule.

And this is just one of countless social rules that must be navigated.

There are numerous ways in which all these rules can be misconstrued and misunderstood. Of immediate concern to a child is anxiety about running afoul of the rules at school, where you can get into trouble with teachers, the principal, and even other students. Some children equate rules with the laws of the land, where infractions will get you in trouble with the police. I have worked with children who think of rules as traps set to catch them. For these children, rules have a negative connotation – always. They are afraid of rules, or rebel against them. Others have a more balanced view. After all, rules can protect you from others – as long as others follow the rules.

On the lighter side, a game has rules in order to define what the game is and to make it fun to play, yet even here there can be anxiety and confusion as all the negative connotations of rules get mixed up with what is supposed to be an enjoyable activity. An Autistic boy has a meltdown when he fails to draw a matching card in a card game. Game rules can in fact feel punitive, and the boy might see himself as bad for "breaking" the match rule when luck doesn't give him the right card. How do you explain? It's not a rule for a person to follow; it's just the rule that says what a match is. One more kind of rule; one more exception to remember.

What happens when nobody explains the rules? Children are often expected to pick up on proper classroom behavior by observing others. Sit quietly in your seat if that's what everyone else is doing. Mingle and interact if that is the format. Play at recess. Be quiet during tests. In other words, *just blend in*. How well does this pan out for a child with a social learning disability who – by definition – cannot pick up on social cues? I think you know the answer. It is no more possible for such a child to unravel the tangle of exceptions for school day behavior than it would be for you to list every possible situation they will ever encounter and teach the appropriate response for each one.

The consequences of breaking rules can be as confusing as the rules themselves. Different rules carry different weights. Driving five miles per hour over the speed limit is very different from sneaking out of a restaurant without paying the bill. Many children on the spectrum have difficulty matching rules with consequences; for them there is no logical pattern to hang on to.

Have you been assuming your child has the same understanding of rules that you do? There are a great many areas for misunderstanding. Watch and listen very carefully to learn how a child views rules. In some cases the concept gaps may be extreme, and adults do little to help. The neurotypical blind spots prevail, and we miss an opportunity to bridge a gap.

Most people don't spend much time thinking about rules in such detail. It all comes rather naturally to neurotypical people, so there's no need to delve into the tangle of exceptions. I'm sure you've noticed by now that the whole point of The Connection Formula is to delve into such things and see them in a new way. After all, you are becoming a confusion detective, and for a child on the spectrum confusion likes to hide in the things we take for granted. Get out your magnifying glass and take a very close look at how your child relates to rules.

Unconfusing the Rules

The Logic of Rules

I suggest that you list some common rules that children encounter and then use the logic scale to see if any seem illogical to your child. Don't do this with an attitude of testing or correcting. Simply explore you child's viewpoint to gain insight into how they perceive things. Make your attitude one of curiosity, compassion and understanding. If it comes to light that your child does not understand a particular rule, validate that yes, rules can be confusing. Then build from there.

When you endeavor to explain a rule, do not make it a lecture. I often use the "did anyone ever tell you" accommodation to explain about rules. Here is an example of how I might address the issue of not acting silly or disruptive during a lesson in the classroom. As you can see in this example, I am not so much focused on the rule itself, which to the child might be just one more arbitrary piece of information to memorize. Instead, I focus on the logic behind the rule in order to put it in context.

👍 *Oh, did anyone ever tell you about teachers? Teachers have over twenty kids in the classroom, and the teacher's brain is filled with the information that they're teaching. It is their job to make sure everyone learns the information that is in the lesson that day. The teacher's mind is so busy with all this information that the teacher is not thinking silly thoughts or fun thoughts. They are thinking informational and educational thoughts.*

Did adults forget to tell you about how a teacher's brain works? Adults are supposed to explain these things!

When a teacher is teaching it is not the best time to be silly because they will not have the time to be silly with you. It is not because they are mean. It is because they are thinking about all the information they have to teach.

I might go on to ask the child, "Who are the silliest adults you know? And who are the serious ones?" I try to keep the conversation going in a direction that does not feel like a lecture.

I present social information as if it is the most interesting new information imaginable, and the children react accordingly, often wide-eyed with amazement that somebody is finally explaining how things are. "You are not like other people," some say. "You always tell the truth,"

Of course I don't believe that other people are lying to these children, but the fact that so many children see it this way is revealing. When a child cannot relate to the social information they are given, it can feel like a lie to them, and trust is lost. So basically, your job is to earn their trust. I'm sure you don't want to be just another adult who hurts their feelings and tells them things that seem senseless and irrelevant. Help them to see the benefit of what you have to offer.

How do you "tell the truth" to an Autistic child? Break down the information, explain the basics, and own the misunderstandings. Try to see things from the child's point of view. Find the connecting logic. Assume that even the most seemingly obvious piece of information will come as a complete revelation to them, because this might very well be so.

These are wonderful moments of connection.

The "What's the Bigger Problem" Game

Ability to prioritize is an important skill, especially when it comes to our relationship with rules. Consider the example at the beginning of this chapter about the child who has a meltdown when the school bus is late. Many children on the spectrum do not like to be late. They consider it a huge, giant, catastrophic problem. However, it is inevitable that everyone will be late sometimes. The lateness problem is not as big as the meltdown problem. Is there a way to start a conversation about this?

To find out how a situation is perceived by a child – and to sneak in some social learning about it – I like to play a game I call *What's the bigger problem?* Here's how it works: pick two problems to compare, and ask your child which problem is bigger. That's it!

I like to "go visual" when I can, so I use a whiteboard when one is available. At the top I write, "What's the bigger problem?" Beneath that I draw a line down the middle of the board. One side is labeled "A"; the other side is "B." Then I write the choices. You don't need to always do it visually, of course, but that's how I'll illustrate the game here.

I generally start with something humorous, or at least something I *think* will be funny. For example:

| What's the bigger problem? ||
| A. Being a cave man chased by a saber tooth tiger. | B. A child forgetting to brush their teeth. |

Be prepared for any response. Some children will laugh and say "A!!!" Other children might realize that problem A will NEVER happen to them and they will pick B. If that happens, you are gaining valuable insights into how they think. You can validate their viewpoint by saying, "Good answer, you are not a cave man and that would never happen to you! So, OBVIOUSLY forgetting to brush your teeth is a more realistic answer. Some people might pretend they are a cave man, and they would have a different answer."

If your child would not see humor in the cave man scenario, then make the choices more relevant to their lives. Don't make questions too scary or put fear into their head.

Here is another light example to get things warmed up. (This is not so light if your child is afraid of either animal that is mentioned, so modify as needed.) This example is more realistic, and therefore more sensitivity is required.

| What's the bigger problem? ||
| A. Finding an ant in the house. | B. Finding the neighbor's cat in the house. |

When you first play this game, try not to correct right away if you feel your child has chosen the wrong priority. Discuss the scenario, and present things in a very neutral way: "Oh, you think an ant is a bigger problem because you like the neighbor's cat. What if the family next door is sad because their cat is missing?"

After some questions along these lines, you can angle toward a problem you wish to address (though I encourage you to play the game even when there is no big problem to solve).

What's the bigger problem?	
A. Dad being five minutes late.	B. You yelling because Dad is five minutes late.

Can you see how that might spark an interesting discussion?

Here are other topics that you might want to address before they become problems:

What's the bigger problem?	
A. Cheating on a test, but passing.	B. Flunking a test.

A. Hitting your brother.	B. Missing your favorite TV show.

Some questions can be about right versus wrong; some about helping a child self-observe; others are just to learn what your child views as important in life.

Some children might not see how the questions are relevant. Fair point. I tell them I like to know how their brain works, because that is interesting to me. "If I know how your brain works then I can understand you better and do more things that your brain might like." Yes, I really do talk this way. Borrow my words, or use your own style.

Very Important Information!

Let's say that Angela is very upset because her sixth birthday is approaching and she believes she will no longer be allowed to play with her five-year-old cousin when they are different ages. This is a very specific misunderstanding of a sort I have seen before. It may have come about at a day camp or during a school activity that divided children by age. How do we handle this effectively?

These factors come into play:

➢ How can we help Angela calm down?

➢ What information will correct the misunderstanding?

➢ How do we give her the information in a way that does not make her feel bad about her mistake?

➢ How can we follow up to make the interaction feel fun and relevant?

With all this in mind, let's ease into a conversation. A possible response to Angela might go something like this:

👍 *Angela, I see there is a BIG problem.*

Hold your hands wide apart while you say this and use a calm, yet exaggerated, tone. The idea is to validate her feelings both with words and gestures.

👍 *I am VERY good at solving problems between 5 year olds and 6 year olds, and I have some VERY IMPORTANT information I forgot to tell you about friendships. I can't wait to tell you my important information and I want your ears to HEAR it.*

At this point pause very briefly and see if you have gotten her attention and calmed her down. If so, you can continue.

👍 *Didn't anyone ever tell you? Five year old and six year old kids can be friends. Friendship rules say that you can be friends with people of lots of different ages if you like each other. I am sooo sorry I forgot to tell you this information before. Does this important information make sense? Yes, no, or I don't know?*

If she accepts the information then you can continue with more. It might be a good time to add the following:

👍 *It is okay to be friends when your parents say it is okay. There is no automatic age limit.*

You can add any other safety related information if you feel it is needed at this time.

The Connection Formula

I sometimes like to ask follow-up questions to keep the conversation going without making things too complicated.

👍 *Who is the oldest person you ever played a game with? What about the times when you play a game with grandma?*

Questions like this are intended to emphasize the topic in a fun way. Don't turn it into a lecture. You can divert toward silliness when things get too serious for a child. "Do you think Grandma is older than six years old? Do you think I am?" Of course if the child misses the humor, hasten to explain. "I am making a joke. I am older than six years old, and grandma is older than me."

When I get into these conversations with children, I always watch their reactions, ready to turn on a dime. You will know your child's sense of humor and their tolerance for serious topics. These techniques can help you know them better.

Correcting the Backstory

There are often many layers to a child's misunderstanding, and I kind of glossed over one in our example of Angela. How did she come to the conclusion that she would not be allowed to play with her cousin if they were different ages? I mentioned that she could have gotten this idea from an activity that separated children by age. How was it that she generalized this one activity into a rule that applied everywhere?

Angela misunderstood the scope of the rule. Nobody explained that the age separation was for one activity only. Who would think they needed to? This is the nature of these concept gaps. The best we can do is spot them early and correct the misunderstanding in a way that feels emotionally safe for the child.

So Angela extrapolated the rule to situations outside the activity. Perhaps the logic was simply easy for her to remember. Maybe it matched her sense of organization, and she found it comforting – that is, until the inevitable consequence of the rule loomed large. The idea of losing a playmate was very upsetting. Erroneous logic was pitted against emotion, and Angela was stuck in the middle.

Of course we might never know exactly how she perceived the situation or how she came to her conclusion. I am making some "what if" guesses here to illustrate how the backstory of these misunderstandings can work. What we do know is that Angela believed the age rule to be a fact, with no possibility that her reasoning could be wrong. In her mind she was 100% certain she would no longer be allowed to play with her cousin. The logic was clearly very appealing to her, even if the result was not. When I uncover a perfectly logical (but wrong) conclusion, I first validate the child's viewpoint, and then try to correct the backstory.

👍 *Your mind is very logical and organized. But there is other information that nobody ever told you...*

Different activities have different rules. Some rules are very logical for one activity, but they do not need to be followed outside the activity. Some rules are for all activities, like not hitting and hurting other people, and some rules are just for that one time, like when the teacher grouped everyone by age.

This can be very confusing! I'm so sorry that adults never explained this to you.

If your child has such difficulties with rules, encourage them to communicate about it. Together you can measure where a rule falls on a logic scale, a safety scale, and a happiness scale. Misunderstood rules will come to light more quickly, and you will be able to help your child understand important rules that they rated low on the logic scale.

Rules, Laws and Guidelines

Sometimes when explaining about rules it is helpful to bring in the idea of laws and guidelines. The tricky part is that the distinction often depends on context.

Let's go back to our discussion about not interrupting. Is it a rule, a law, or a guideline? In most situations it is certainly not a law – you will not get arrested for interrupting a conversation at party. But it's quite a different story in a courtroom, where interrupting the judge has much more serious consequences. And it's more of a guideline in the situations your child normally encounters, although there are times when it becomes a rule. Are you allowed to interrupt when talking to friends? As a guideline we say it's not polite, yet it happens all the time and usually it's no big deal (unless it happens too frequently). Now what about a school play – can you just stand up and ask a question? The rule says no, do not interrupt a performance – and it's kind of strict.

Does your child understand this? Do they know the difference between a rule and a guideline? Do they know that the difference may depend on who they are interacting with? Here is one of those countless concepts that we take for granted. The rules are relaxed among friends, tend to become stricter among strangers, and become stricter still when dealing with structured events (like an assembly or church) or authority figures (your teacher, your boss, and certainly authorities like the police). An Autistic child will not necessarily be aware of these distinctions, so you will need to break down the information. Explain about rules, laws and guidelines.

Agreements, Negotiations and Promises

If you can find connecting logic to something your child considers reasonable it will make rules seem more fair and less arbitrary. Along these lines, it can be helpful to present a family rule as an agreement:

👍 *I agree to plan the dinner, shop for the groceries, cook the dinner, and have it ready at 6:00pm. You agree to come to the dinner table at six o'clock. Does that seem fair?*

Some children on the spectrum don't understand why parents get to make non-negotiable decisions. Your child may need to be taught the difference between what is negotiable and what is not. School, of course, is not negotiable:

👍 *All children in this country need to get an education. That is the law. Therefore, I need to make sure you learn. That is my job.*

Unconfusing the Rules

At home you may find plenty of opportunities for negotiation. Perhaps your child has drawn something on a whiteboard and doesn't want to erase it – ever. To negotiate, offer logical alternatives:

👍 *I have an idea: we can take a picture of your drawing and put it on the computer. Then we can print the picture and put it on the wall. Is that a good idea? Can we erase the whiteboard after we take the picture?*

If your child agrees, then your agreement is a promise. You have to print the picture and put it on the wall. When you make a promise, your child may see it as a rule. I encourage the use of promises – *if* they can be kept.

Child-Empowering Rules

Some children have told me that they feel like a slave because their parents always tell them what to do. There is an effective way to balance this: come up with some rules that have an upside for your child. Show them what's in it for them. This helps remove negative connotations from the concept of rules. For example, you may agree that each family member can choose the meal once a week. This is a fun rule that parents commit to, and it has a clear upside to the child when it's their turn to chose. It is like a promise.

I really like to use rules that show a commitment to a child. This allows you to become more reliable and dependable in their eyes. When you make a mutual agreement that binds you to a promise, you are showing that the system can work both ways, and that rules are not arbitrary and one-sided. (Obviously you need to follow through on the promise, or you have defeated the purpose.)

In a similar vein, I have allowed children in my socialization groups to create rules that express their own goals. They added "have fun" as a rule, posted on the wall with all the others. I adhere to it as much as possible. This particular rule sparks many interesting and thought-provoking discussions.

I call these *child-empowering rules*. Begin introducing them early. They help remove the negative connotations of rules, and provide the groundwork for socialization outside the home.

When we get to Family Fun Time in the Socialization part of the book, it will be very important to have some rules in place in order to maximize the chance of success. To be clear, please do not think of this as a way to force your child to behave a certain way. That misses the heart of The Connection Formula, and it will surely take away the fun. A child who is nervous about socializing does not need to be made more nervous by a long list of rules to follow.

Instead, present the rules as useful social information. These rules should ease your child's mind about what is expected and what may or may not happen. Here are the kind of rules I'm talking about:

- Parents will demonstrate activities before asking children to do them.
- Parents lead the activities and will decide who goes first.
- Parents might make mistakes in explaining an activity, but they are not doing it on purpose.
- You can correct Mom or Dad and they will not get mad.
- Watching an activity before participating is fine.
- "I don't know" is an okay answer.
- Everything on the schedule does not need to be accomplished.
- Have fun!
- There will be more fun time tomorrow.

These rules have a different feeling to them, don't they? They are there to support fun in a child-relatable way, and are not used as an obvious boundary for bad behavior. They make life predictable for the child and ensure that everyone has similar expectations regarding the flow of activities. It is this philosophy, the feeling behind the rules, that makes a big difference.

Unconfusing the Rules

Some rules about behavior are necessary, of course. Even these rules can be presented in a child-empowering way. Just think about the social norms behind the rule, and then convey the rule as a piece of social information. For example, here are some rules about talking:

➢ Ideas don't all need to be said out loud.

➢ If you have something to say when other people are talking, then you can write it on a whiteboard.

➢ Repeat the same joke no more than three times. After that it is not funny.

When presented in this way, rules can cover a lot of ground without negative connotations. There is an upside for the child. Some rules will still sound like plain old rules, of course, and it is fine to sprinkle in "classic" rules like these:

➢ Ask before touching people or things.

➢ No bullying.

The goal is for your child to learn to see the mutual social benefit behind rules, so that they do not all seem entirely arbitrary and illogical. Your child will encounter plenty of rules outside of an environment that you control – and some of these rules are, indeed, arbitrary and illogical. Others are completely specious, such as a bully's admonition not to tattle. Bullies don't get to make the rules. Your child will have much to learn.

The way you present rules at home can go a long way toward overcoming emotional resistance to the topic. The key is to introduce rules a little at a time, presenting them in an empowering and logical manner.

The rules I've presented are just examples, so you're going to need time to figure out what is needed for your child. If you present a big list of rules all at once – no matter how child-friendly and empowering you make them – I can guarantee it will be confusing to your child *and* to you. You won't have enough information to know what works, and your child will wonder what is going on with this new way of engaging with you. So don't change everything at once. Sprinkle these ideas into normal routines. Child-empowering rules are accommodations that should be introduced long before you get to more advanced work like Family Fun Time and play date planning, where rules and structure become even more of a focus.

Take things one step at a time. You won't know enough in the beginning to predict where you will end up. Ease into socialization and you will have the best chance of success.

16

Problem Solving

Problem solving can be quite an interesting journey when dealing with Autistic children, or any child for that matter. The more a child and adult are on the same page – in other words, the more we share a mutual understanding about the world and each other – the better the chance of success.

What kinds of problems are we trying to solve? Pretty much anything that comes up in daily life: misunderstandings, conflicts with siblings, bad surprises, homework difficulties...the list is long. We don't want to deal with each problem as a one-off emergency. It is best to have a system in place. A problem solving system is comforting for your child *and* for you. The very idea of problems can be filled with stress. We want to reduce the stress, soothe a child's anxiety, and make their life – and yours – more predictable. Instead of feeling panic (*oh no, not another problem!*) we want the family to feel a sense of purpose (*ah, now we get to use our problem solving system*). That is a challenging goal, but quite worth the effort. Any step in this direction will make life a little bit easier.

Now I have to address the overarching problem that always seems to trump our careful plans: the problem of behavior. The neurotypical view of autism puts behavior front and center. That is the big problem that gets all the attention, and yes, it is a huge concern. I have steered you away from a direct assault on behavior problems because, without the right starting point, you won't get the best result...and you may do more harm than good. Behavior isn't the real problem. It's a symptom.

The real problem is the challenge of building reciprocal communication, which we have been working on all along.

The Behavior Breadcrumb Trail

Let's look at that phrase: "behavior problem." Behavior refers to your child's way of being in the world. If a child's way of being is a problem for you and others, then something very deep is going on within the child. That is the real problem we're trying to understand.

When you're too steeped in traditional thinking, behavior won't give you a proper hint of what the real problem is. It's easy to think you know where the breadcrumb trail leads, so you follow false markers to a wrong conclusion. In truth, behavior is often evidence of something deeper. The trail we want to follow does not lead to pat answers; it leads instead to important questions...*what if* style questions. And what do you need to get your answers? Accommodations. Trust. Reciprocal communication.

How can two people see the same behavior and be led in such different directions? It depends on what you're looking for. One mindset looks for a way to control behavior; the other looks for misunderstandings, concept gaps, sensory issues...anything that leads to true insight and a child who feels safe and understood.

Reciprocal communication is the starting point for an effective problem solving system. As you and your child gain confidence in your ability to communicate, you can at last begin to dig out problems at the root. This approach is proactive in the extreme because it builds a foundation for dealing with all manner of problems in an expansive way. Each success builds momentum.

First Connect

Fortunately you don't need to have an immediate solution for every problem that arises. Simply validating that the problem exists is a giant step in the right direction. It connects you and your child.

Problem validation builds on the running commentary technique described in Chapter 6. The goal is to state the problem in a way that acknowledges your child's point of view. However, you cannot assume

Problem Solving

that you really understand your child's viewpoint, so it is best to stick to very literal facts. Remember, facts are comforting.

Also, sticking with facts minimizes the chance of "validating" the wrong thing, adding confusion instead of reducing it. Believe me, I have added confusion in plenty of problem solving sessions. What do I do? I own the mistake, then try to keep the conversation going by looking for a more accurate way to state the problem according to the child's view of it.

Here are some examples of problem validation statements. Notice how they use literal facts and try to avoid assumptions.

👍 *Oh, I understand that you don't want to do your homework.*

👍 *Your sister and you want to watch different TV shows.*

👍 *Your brother is talking at the same time you are talking.*

👍 *The toast got burned and you don't like burned toast.*

👍 *Your favorite pants are too small for you now because you grew.*

With this type of validation we keep things very simple and literal. Freeze the moment, take a mental snapshot of it, and state what's going on in a way your child relates to. If you don't slow yourself down like this, you may jump to conclusions and not know it.

We start with extremely basic validations so we can begin to compare and contrast our viewpoint with the child's view of the world:

👍 *I see you want to play your video game when I am telling you to go to bed.*

Stating the problem in a literal way helps you discover what the problem really is. The tone here should be reassuring, showing that you understand your child's point of view.

If you find that despite your best efforts you still have not hit on the child's viewpoint, back up and try again.

👍 *Oh, I think that bedtime came when you were about to reach a new level in your video game.*

In my profession, I have to correct myself all the time. I've had an enormous amount of practice weeding out assumptions and breaking things down into literal statements. Even so, I do not always get it right the first time. There will always be trial and error involved. I often find myself telling children, "I made a mistake with my words." Then I go on to restate the problem in light of what I learn from the child's reaction. You will get to know your own child better through this process. It's not important to always be right. It is important to always be flexible.

A child may learn to use accommodations independently to explain their problem to you. Here, too, validating statements are important.

Your child says they are "substitute teacher nervous" about the new neighbors. Here is a validating response:

👍 *It's not fun to be nervous like when the substitute teacher came.*

Your child points to Level 4 on the safety scale. You can reply:

👍 *I don't want you to have a Level 4. I want to change things so that it can be a one or a two.*

Your child says that the someone being mean at recess is a bigger problem than breaking the law. A response like this offers comfort and support:

👍 *I'm so sorry that someone was mean to you at recess. We need to solve this problem about mean people!*

Do you get the idea? Whether or not you feel a problem is a big one for *you*, try to honor the problem as seen through your child's eyes. This means having no judgment. Putting validation first will also help to slow down the communication, taking the stress out of it.

Validation is just as important when your child begins to participate

Problem Solving

in problem solving and contribute their own ideas. It's important to validate their contributions, even if you need to redirect them.

👍 *That is a good idea. Your mind is working well. Here is another idea.*

If you hold the intention of being a patient and sensitive problem solver, you will naturally begin to validate your child's viewpoint. Validation begins to get the problem on the table. You obviously need the right view of the problem before you can solve it.

Getting the Problem on the Table

For a child on the spectrum, the root of a problem is not always obvious. You need to get the problem on the table and illuminate how your child perceives the situation without judging or immediately trying to fix it. Sometimes a simple solution will present itself just by bringing out the facts.

Let's see how this can play out. What follows is an example showing what it might take to get a homework problem on the table.

The Impossible Homework

Let's say that Sebastian has become very upset at homework time, and does not want to do the work. His parents tried a direct approach and asked exactly what the homework assignment was, but Sebastian became even more agitated and replied, "I told you it's IMPOSSIBLE!" When a direct approach is upsetting to a child, it's time to go to the accommodations.

Validate	Parent: "You told me that the homework is impossible. That does sound like a problem."
Use a problem scale	Parent: "How big is the impossible problem?" Sebastian indicates that it's a BIG problem in wide part of the problem pyramid.

Well, we already knew it was a big problem due to his emotional state. Going to the problem pyramid or a 1-5 scale helps slow things

The Connection Formula

down, and might help calm him. And in any case, it is best to double check. Never assume. Always gather your data.

<u>Validate</u>	Parent: "Now I know the homework problem is a big problem, thank you for showing me."
<u>Break it down into steps</u>	Here the parent uses a walkthrough of the homework timeline, bouncing around a bit to pinpoint the problem.
	Parent: "When I say 'It's time to do homework,' is that a big problem?"
	Sebastian: "Yes."
	Parent: "If you sit down at your desk and start to do your homework, is that a big problem?"
	Sebastian: "Yes"
	Parent: "Was bringing the homework home with you a big problem?"
	Sebastian: "No."
	Parent: "Was getting the homework from your teacher a big problem?"
	Sebastian: "YES!"
<u>Validate</u>	Parent: "It was a big problem when your teacher gave you the homework. It is not good that you have a big problem."
<u>Give concrete choices</u>	Parent: "You have homework in math and spelling. Is spelling a big problem, yes or no?"
	Sebastian: "Spelling is not a big problem."
<u>Validate</u>	Parent: "When the teacher gave you the math homework it was a big problem."

Sebastian: "Yes."

Think *what if*	Here his parent just makes a guess.
	Parent: "Was the teacher wrong to give you the homework?"
	Sebastian: "Yes."
	Now we may be getting somewhere…
Mix in compliments	Parent: "You are very good at math. This must be a VERY interesting problem!"
	Sebastian: "It's IMPOSSIBLE."
Use the logic scale	Parent: "Show me how impossible on the logic scale."
	Sebastian indicates 5: *This makes no sense.*
Validate	Parent: "The math problem does not make sense."
	Sebastian: "The math problem DOES make sense. The answer is eight."
Own the misunderstanding	Parent: "Oh, that is my mistake. The problem makes sense, but the homework does not make sense."

Are we getting somewhere or not? The parent's statement does not make much sense…to the *parent*. It does seem to make sense to Sebastian. He is calm, perhaps enjoying the process because he's being heard.

Confirm by other accommodations	With the logic scale, the parent learns that the math problem is Level 1: Very Logical.
	The homework assignment, however, is a Level 5. It makes no sense to Sebastian.

The Connection Formula

With this confirmation, it's time to break things down some more and get to the bottom of the paradox.

<u>Break down into steps</u>

Parent: "Did the teacher tell you how to do the homework?"

Sebastian: "Yes."

Parent: "Did she teach you how to do the math?"

Sebastian: "I KNOW how to do the math. She said to draw the trees."

And another piece falls into place. Drawing trees is part of the math homework!

<u>Validate</u>

Parent: "Drawing tress when you do your math homework is a big problem."

Sebastian: "Yes, I can't draw all the trees."

<u>Break down into steps</u>

Parent: "Is it a big problem to draw a tree?"

Sebastian: "No. I can draw a tree."

Parent: "Is it a big problem drawing more than one tree?"

Sebastian: "I need to draw ten divided by two trees and then add three. The answer is eight. But I can only draw FIVE trees on the paper. I'm going to get the answer WRONG."

<u>Validate</u>

Parent: "You know the answer is eight, but you can only draw five trees. That is very confusing for a good math student like you."

Sebastian: "The teacher said to draw them for homework, but I CAN'T."

<u>Conclusion</u>: The parent knows Sebastian has problems with visual/spatial relations, and thinks, *he probably drew five big trees and*

then there was no space for three more. I can tell him that all eight trees do not need to be the same size.

This seems like a long road to a simple solution. However, the true problem here was not about drawing trees for a math problem. It was about a concept gap that led a child to believe he was dealing with an impossible task, and his emotional readiness to handle the resulting stress and confusion.

The true solution was not the conclusion (draw smaller trees); it was the process itself. The process keeps the child calm. It keeps you calm. It allows you to discover the source of a child's anxiety, which is usually due to a missing concept or a neurologically different way of viewing things. The specifics vary greatly, but when a child is on the autism spectrum, the impact of this neurological difference is important to uncover in any problem you are trying to solve.

If you focus solely on reaching a quick conclusion, you'll miss the relevance of the process. Break things down into very small steps, both for the child's benefit and your own. Yes, breaking things down into steps helps *you*. It creates space to consider what might be going on in your child's thought process. It gives you the opportunity to find the concept gaps and enlighten yourself about how your child sees things. That won't happen when you're moving too fast; you'll miss the scenery, so to speak. You won't see your child's thought process if your steps are too big. You'll glide right past connection points if you're too focused on correcting.

Big steps have blind spots. You need to look for small steps in the gaps between the big ones, where you never thought to look before.

Minimize Stress

Some children are not able to keep sustained attention on problems for more than a minute or so. It is just too stressful. Stress makes it hard to face a problem and solve it; the problem then becomes bigger than the child's coping strategies. An effective problem solving system will decrease your child's stress.

Do not force your child into long problem solving interactions if it causes them distress. If there is a feeling of conflict, proceed cautiously. If the negative feeling peaks quickly and leads to a sense of mutual cooperation, then you are on the right track. On the other hand, if the problem solving strategies in this chapter do not calm your child and you feel you need some help, then you might consider finding a qualified counselor.

The more you are seen as a successful problem solver, the more confidence your child will have in you, and that is VERY important. Now here's the catch: when *you* are stressed out it is hard to calmly address a situation; it feels overwhelming, and who wants to keep sustained attention on *that* feeling? Calm communication is the key to effective problem solving.

We need to minimize stress in everyone.

Make a Plan to Make a Plan

Let's say a child demands your attention when you are very busy. See if you can identify what is wrong with the following response:

👎 *I know you're frustrated because I can't talk to you right now, but you'll have to wait."*

Is this response simple enough? Does this create a space for understanding between you and the child? I would say no. This statement makes too many assumptions and does not create space for anything. For example, the child might not actually be frustrated, or might not know the word relates to their feelings. There are just too many big concepts thrown in together.

How about this one:

👎 *You are being impatient right now."*

I find this sort of statement to be unhelpful because it's all about *your* point of view. It is far too critical and shows little understanding of the child. Not validating at all.

Here is a good response that is validating and reassuring:

👍 *You have something important to discuss with me and you need me to listen and answer. I do want to answer. In ten minutes we will make a plan to solve your problem. Solving your problem is very important to me.*

This response does something very helpful: it presents a plan – a *plan to make a plan.* You don't need an answer in the moment. As simple as this is, it can be a life saver for some children.

Be Specific and Concrete

One Autistic child I know has a "parent dictionary" in his head. He told me, "When my parents say 'we'll see,' they mean 'no.'" Would his parents recognize his definition? It's hard to say. *We'll see* is one of countless vague responses about the future. We all use such expressions: *Later, not now, I'll think about it, maybe, it depends...* Neurotypical people have little problem with these expressions because we understand context and body language, whereas a child on the autism spectrum can easily miss these clues. Each child is left on their own to guess the meaning.

Often *we'll see* is a parent's way of saying, "we'll talk about it later." But what does the expression mean in a literal sense? What will we see? And when exactly will we see it? If you look at it this way, it's more than a little bit vague. There is no literal information for a child to hang on to.

For many children on the spectrum, a vague response is not a rational response. So let's think in specifics. A child asks if he can go to the movies. Instead of saying *we'll see,* try being more concrete. Make a plan to make a plan:

👍 *It is fun to go to the movies. I will have to look on the calendar to see where it fits there. We have many fun things to do. I promise we will make a plan before Friday.*

It is okay not to have an answer in the moment. The more definite you can be about a timeline, the more comfortable your child will be:

👍 *I don't know now. I have to talk with your father first to see if his schedule is free. I will have an answer by three o'clock.*

Always give a specific time, whether it's later that afternoon or later in the week. Don't just leave a problem hanging.

👍 *We will talk about it in one hour.*

👍 *I will give you an answer when I pick you up at school.*

👍 *It is hard for me to answer while I change the baby. I will answer after dinner.*

Note that these statements are very specific and concrete, and that's exactly what is needed. Make your comments measurable, quantifiable, and specific about time. It is a way of talking which might not come naturally at first, but it's a valuable skill to develop. For many Autistic children it's comforting to have a concrete plan in place, even if that plan is to make a plan later.

Validate, Explain, Arrange

If you're tempted to say *we'll see* (or any such vague expression), stop and think about what you mean in that moment. You probably mean that you don't have time to stop and think! Fair enough, you can't answer the question right now. Is there any specific information you *can* give? What do you literally mean by *we'll see*?

Perhaps you mean something like this:

👎 *I have no idea how to answer you because I am making dinner and watching the baby at the same time and can't even think about the next five minutes, never mind the next few hours. I'm going to burn dinner if I put any attention on this. My multitasking is maxed out!*

If that's the case, then an answer like this might be more helpful:

👍 *You asked a good question. My mind has five thoughts in it right now and it is filled. I will answer it while we eat dinner. Dinner is in fifteen minutes.*

This type of answer does three things:

- ➢ It validates the question.

- ➢ It explains what is happening in the moment by giving concrete information about it.

- ➢ It arranges an action plan with a specific time frame.

I have trained myself to answer questions in this fashion, gearing my response to the specific child. It is well worth learning how to validate, explain, and arrange a time for action.

I always start with a validating statement. It connects with the child – and it gives me a second or two to think of what I'm going to say next! Here are a few more examples:

👍 *Watching a movie will be fun.*

👍 *Knowing the schedule is important.*

👍 *I'm glad you asked that question.*

Next, I explain some social information, based on the child's ability to understand. Some children will understand the implications if you say, "My mind has five thoughts in it right now." Others might not. In this case, you can explain a little more:

👍 *While I am cooking I will think of an answer. It will take longer to think of an answer because I am doing five things at once. It is hard for me so I cannot answer you right now.*

Finally, it's important to arrange a concrete action plan. Offer a plan along these lines:

👍 *Write the question down and put it in the question bowl and we'll review it after dinner.*

The Connection Formula

👍 *Write down three movies you would like to watch and after dinner we will choose which one to watch.*

👍 *Draw a picture of a character from the movie and show it to me while we eat dinner.*

👍 *Set the timer for fifteen minutes and ask me again when the timer goes off.*

As you give concrete information, learn to be patient with the responses you get as your child tries to make sense of your words. For example, if you bring up the question while serving brownies after the meal, some children might say, "You lied to me, you said we would talk about it during dinner, and brownies are not dinner, they are dessert!"

Children on the autism spectrum are not necessarily trying to be contrary; they are simply trying to make sense of the situation. Literal information provides anchor points, and when those anchor points change arbitrarily, their world is thrown into chaos – literally. The best sort of response in this situation is to simply own the mistake:

👍 *That's a good point. I made a mistake with my words. I meant to say dessert, not dinner.*

A child also might ask for specific details, such as what five things are in your head. What do I do when children press me for details? I give them details! Pick five concrete things, for example: 1. cooking hamburgers, 2. steaming vegetables, 3. making a salad, 4. setting the table, and 5. watching your sister. (And be glad you didn't say there were *fifty* things in your head! Exaggeration does not exactly work well with a literal communication style.)

The more you use concrete phrases and specific information, the more your child will feel safe and understood. As your child feels less confused, you will be able to shorten some of this concrete information. It is easier to see when and where miscommunication occurs when the language is concrete. It makes the communication process more visible.

Problem Solving

The following table gives some more ideas on how to validate, explain and arrange. Mix and match – and of course fill in your own specifics. In time you'll find the best way of validating your child; these examples are to get you started.

Validate	Explain	Arrange
You asked a good question.	My mind is busy trying to solve another problem.	We will talk about it after dinner.
I like the way your brain works.	It is hard for me to answer while I change the baby.	I will answer you in one hour.
That is a very interesting question.	I need time to think of a good answer.	I will give you an answer when I pick you up at school.
That sounds like a big problem.	You sister is sick and needs my attention. It's hard for me to do two things at the same time.	Go write the problem on the whiteboard and I will come get you when I am done with your sister.
Answering that question is important to me.	We want to have a lot of time to talk about it, but now it is almost bedtime. We need 30 minutes to talk about it, and bedtime is in five minutes.	Write down the question and put it in the problem jar. Our next "problem jar time" is tomorrow when you get home from school. Then we will have time to talk about it.
That is a good idea you have for Saturday.	We have many other fun things planned that day.	Tonight I will look on the calendar to see if it fits on Saturday.

The Connection Formula

You won't be able to talk this way all the time, but if you do enough of it your child will begin to feel more comfortable. Once children know you're able to be literal when they need you to be, they are much happier. There's a trust that begins to form.

The Problem Jar

When your child comes to you with a problem, it is important to handle it as thoroughly as possible. It may require too much time to address each problem on the fly throughout the day, so you make a plan to make a plan. This is where a problem jar can work wonders. Of course you can use a box or a basket or any type of container. You can let your child decorate it by writing a label or drawing a picture.

The problem jar provides a space and place for a child to share problems and seek your help to find solutions. It is a way for children to learn how to identify their problems and concerns. Your child puts a problem in the jar, and you schedule time to help solve it. It is a way for you to remember to keep your promise when the pace of the day does not allow you to solve a problem as soon as it comes up. The jar is therefore part of a definitive plan for identifying and addressing problems. It can be used for problems that arise at home, in school, or pretty much anywhere.

Without a problem jar you might not even realize that your child has a problem. Giving your child a place to put problems gives you more insight into their life. Handling problems from the jar clarifies misunderstandings and creates a better dictionary of communication between you and your child.

One format for using a problem jar is to make problem slips using the 1-5 scales or the problem pyramid, depending on your child's preference. Print multiple copies per page and cut them out. Keep a supply of these near the problem jar, in your purse, or at pre-determined places in the house. (The problem scales need to be pre-taught so your child is already comfortable with them before you introduce this new way to use them.)

When there is a problem, your child can take one of the slips and add the pertinent information. Have them circle the level on the 1-5 scale or mark the level on the problem pyramid. That much may be easy. Describing the problem can be more difficult. Simply writing down when or where the problem occurred may be sufficient: *Recess problem. Playground problem.* Or you can suggest labeling the problem with a title so your child doesn't feel the need to write down all the details. Think of it as the title of a story: *Need a New Bicycle. Homework Help. The Ripped Science Book.* Something short – the details can wait until later. Help your child write this on the back of the slip. (Eventually they may be able to do it independently.) The problem slip is then placed in the jar.

That is the first part of the process. Now a time needs to be scheduled for reviewing the problems in the jar. A specific daily time is best. It is important to respect and honor the scheduled review time. Treat it like a promise. Your child might not remind you, but that doesn't mean they do not see the process as important. It can be comforting for some children to know that they will not have to remind you.

It is very useful to consider the problem ahead of time, not only to come up with a solution, but also to plan ways to present the solution to your child. Decide ahead of time which accommodations are appropriate. I've had a good deal of practice improvising in the moment; even so, I like to have a plan, a backup plan, and a backup plan for the backup plan. The Connection Formula works best when you think proactively about the interactions with your child, perhaps a lot more than you're used to. Don't worry, though; it's something you grow into. When you consistently use accommodations, this level of proactive planning usually requires just a few moments of thought...depending, of course, on the nature of the problem.

By the way, the problem jar is not just for problems. It can also be used for deferred decisions. For example, your child may ask to go the library on Saturday. It is only Wednesday, you are cooking dinner and the phone is ringing. In this case you can ask your child to fill out a slip and put it in the jar. The description of the problem might be *Library on Saturday*.

Parent Request Forms

Sometimes I suggest using a "parent request form" if these scenarios come up frequently. Just as you involved your child in decorating the problem jar, you can enlist their help in

> designing a form that they can use to write down their request. The request can go in the jar, or you can use another container, like an envelope on the refrigerator. I have even found toy mailboxes for this purpose. The child puts the flag up when they have "mailed" a request.
>
> Of course you understand that this idea of writing down problems and requests is not to put some kind of formal bureaucratic barrier between you and your child. Quite the opposite: the process builds trust. It gives your child a concrete anchor point and makes life in the family more predictable and comfortable. Whatever system you put in place should be reassuring to them.

I know many families who have created a problem jar and never used it. It is your job to use it consistently, even if your child does not remind you. Any time you try something new give it about a month before giving up on the idea. If an idea doesn't work right away, I encourage you to adapt it to meet the needs of your family. For example, you can use sticky notes or scrap paper instead of printing the problem scales. Just please don't give up on an idea too soon.

A Plan Is a Promise

You cannot always drop everything to immediately focus on a problem, but you can always validate that the problem exists, and then make a plan to create a plan later. Let me illustrate the importance of following through.

Say Gabe, your nine year old, says that he is "thunderstorm scared" about going to visit grandma on Saturday. You know from working with feeling phrases that *thunderstorm* refers to a big scary problem for him. What do you do? Well, if he brings up the problem while you are driving to the doctor's office because your three year old has an ear infection and she is screaming in the back seat, then this is hardly the ideal time to create a plan about the weekend visit. You can say:

👍 *Thunderstorm sacred is a BIG problem. Your sister has a big problem too. I am a good problem solver. First I will solve your sister's prob-*

lem, and before you go to bed tonight we will write down your problem about grandma. Tomorrow we will make a solution to the "grandma thunderstorm" problem after you come home from school and before you start homework.

This is a good start. Making a plan to create a plan is a very concrete way to validate your child's feelings. Of course you can't just let it stop there. The plan is a promise, and you must keep your promises to keep your child's trust.

Gabe might not remind you about the grandma problem, so it is your job to remember. Gabe may think, "Okay, now I don't need to think about the grandma problem, Mom will solve it." What happens when Saturday rolls around and it is time for the visit with grandma? Gabe never mentioned it again, so you just let it go. Now you are walking up the driveway to grandma's house when the friendly neighbor waves and says, "Hi, it's nice to see you again – I just made some cookies and will drop them off."

And suddenly Gabe has a major meltdown.

Uh-oh. Could this have something to do with the "thunderstorm scared" problem that you never followed up on?

Let's go back in time. Last week during a visit, this same neighbor brought over cookies with an aroma that Gabe could not tolerate. (It might have been quite pleasant for everyone else, like cinnamon or ginger.) It was just too much for his senses to manage, so Gabe ran into the back yard. No one knew why or even gave it a second thought, and Gabe did not have the words to explain about his sensitivity.

Back to the present. Gabe sees the neighbor and can still imagine that horrific smell. Now he experiences something like this: "Mom you NEVER solved the problem, you said you would and now the problem is here again!!!"

Saying all that is too hard, but the feeling is still there. It is as if Mom completely let him down. She did not help solve the problem and can't be relied on. He tried his best to advocate for himself on the car ride to the doctor's office, and it didn't work. Gabe might conclude that going to visit grandma is just not worth the effort. He also might conclude that his family just can't help him with his day-to-day life. And would he be completely wrong?

The Connection Formula

The size of his disappointment may be reflected in the scale of the meltdown. I hope you see this is not just about the aroma of cookies, or whatever the particular issue happens to be. It is about your child having someone to trust to make life feel stable and safe.

I know it's not always easy to remember everything you say to your child – especially when your focus is elsewhere – but it's very important to make sure you don't break your promises. Remember to follow up on them. That alone will allow your child to feel safe and understood. This is why tools like the problem jar are very important.

Creating a "Bad Surprise" Plan

What is a bad surprise? It is an unwelcome event. You can pretty much assume that any change from a child's expectations is going to fall into this category. Change can be disorienting and scary. How do you deal with it? Plan ahead for bad surprises. Introduce the plan in calm moments, then execute quickly when there is an unexpected change.

First, teach what a bad surprise is. Don't assume that your child knows about surprises, good or bad. They might know the word, but it's important to connect it to personal experience. Usually there will be plenty of bad surprise examples to choose from.

👍 *You like to play your video game after doing homework, but one day the electricity went out in a storm. That is a bad surprise.*

Draw upon any such past experience to pre-teach what a bad surprise is. This builds your child's vocabulary for feelings. If you have some feeling phrases in place, it should be easy to find one that helps illustrate a bad surprise.

Have a bad surprise plan at the ready. For example, have three things in mind that will be fun for your child. (Buying their favorite action figure; adding a half an hour of game time; making their favorite dessert.) If a bad surprise occurs, substitute one or more of the three things instead. Obviously these are very child-specific. Some children will like to watch a movie. Others might prefer a visit to the library.

Does this sound like a plan to balance disappointment with treats and rewards? Well, there is that aspect to it. However, an Autistic child's experience of a bad surprise has implications beyond disappointment. A bad surprise is disorienting. It can make the world seem unpredictable, as if cause and effect cannot be trusted. So we are doing more than softening the disappointment. We are grounding the child's experience to show that the world has not spun off its axis. We are teaching that bad surprises happen, and when they do, we will have a plan. Cause and effect is restored.

Explain the bad surprise plan. Now you need to introduce this whole idea to your child.

👍 *If a bad surprise happens, we will do these three things...*

Keep the list handy; bring it with you on outings. Show the list to your child to make it concrete.

Execute the plan when a bad surprise occurs. Out comes the list. Use an emphatic, calm, and confident tone of voice to convey that everything is under control.

👍 *This is a bad surprise! Now it is time to use our bad surprise plan. We get to do these three things that are fun in place of the bad surprise.*

Sometimes you will need to add specific social information about the situation. For example, let's say that you promised ice cream after errands but the ice cream stand is closed by the time you get there. How disappointing this is for anyone! But from the neurotypical viewpoint, it does not mean the loss of all ice cream in the world. You might need to explain this to an Autistic child:

👍 *Ice cream still exists. You will have ice cream again. Do you want to make a plan for when you will have ice cream?*

Now do the bad surprise plan, make a new ice cream plan, or both.

Bad Surprise Tokens

Here's another idea: Give your child a "bad surprise token" when a bad surprise occurs. The token is "redeemable" by your child for a favorite treat, movie, or purchase. You can use different colored tokens for different levels of a bad surprise. This might lead to a helpful discussion about the level of "badness" of the surprise. It normalizes the idea that sometimes plans change unexpectedly, and helps a child navigate the emotional sting of the disappointment.

Consider making the tokens redeemable for items from a "bad surprise prize box" at home. The box could contain small items and/or written promises: *We will go to a movie. You can buy a new puzzle book.* Be creative, and bring your child in on the plan. Enlist their help to decide on the prizes, decorate the prize box, or color the tokens. And of course, *always* honor the promise represented by the token.

Without a bad surprise plan, parents are forced to improvise. There's a scramble to make an alternate plan. Will you be able to calm your child down? Too much attention on emotions can stress an Autistic child even more. Having a plan in place puts the focus on something other than your child – it puts the focus on the plan.

A bad surprise is a big opportunity. We try to do more than just calm a child in the moment. We make the world safe, and that creates an opening for us to teach them how to tolerate strong emotions.

Transitions and Waiting Activities

Transitions are changes, whether large or small. Some are barely noticeable to us, like turning the page in a book. (I call these micro-transitions, and we will meet them again in Chapter 20.) Others are very big and obvious, such as going on vacation, transitioning from middle school to high school, or moving to a new town. In between there are transitions we experience often: driving from one place to another, changing topics in a conversation, a change in schedule or routine, and countless more.

All transitions can be challenging and confusing for someone on the autism spectrum. With big transitions you are not likely to miss the need for big preparation. What about those in-between transitions? I'm especially thinking of transitions that keep you waiting unexpectedly: a traffic jam, a crowded waiting room, slow service at a restaurant, a long check-out line at the grocery store...nobody likes these bad surprises. Face it: we can pretty much expect an "unexpected" delay at any time. Do we bother to prepare for them? Things can go much more smoothly if you do.

I will often make up questions in the moment to help a child through small transitions. For example, what is it like for your child while you are putting groceries in the trunk or securing their sibling in the car seat? Be sensitive to these moments; the very concept of waiting may be unclear. Here is a great chance to head off confusion with a waiting activity:

👍 *Look for green cars in the parking lot while I buckle in your sister.*

This gives information on what is going on and helps your child know what to do before they find themselves confused by a transition.

Some children on the autism spectrum find waiting to be nearly intolerable unless we have a strategy to ease them through. Waiting activities are very important and can be used during a variety of transitions. If you plan ahead you can have activity books, electronic games, and other supplies available to keep your child occupied. But these are not always practical; and besides, our goal is not to keep your child continuously absorbed in solitary activities. It's nice to have some interactive fun to keep communication going between the two of you. Fortunately, many interactive activities can be carried in your head, like observation questions, trivia questions, and guessing games.

Here are some ideas. Adjust for your child's age, abilities, and interests.

➢ How many chairs are in this waiting room?

➢ How many blue things do you see?

➢ How many foods can you list that are the color red?

The Connection Formula

- How many grocery carts are in this aisle?
- How many grocery items do we have? Count as we put them on the check-out conveyor belt.
- Does the person in front of us have any of the things we have in our cart?
- Are people wearing sneakers or another type of shoe?
- Guess the animal: "I have stripes, they are black and white, I am from Africa." (Zebra)

> There are many online trivia games that can help you. For example, apps can be downloaded onto your phone so you can play animal sounds. Or make the sounds yourself!

- Guess the TV character: "I live under the sea. My best friend is pink. I have yellow pants." (SpongeBob).

Give bigger hints if your child is confused by the clues.

- Use your child's special interests for a spontaneous trivia game:
  - Can you name three facts about World War II?
  - Name three buildings you have been to that have escalators.
  - Can you quote four different lines from The Simpsons?
  - Name four Disney movies, and one character from each movie.
- Try the "copy me" game:
  - Clap your hands twice, and ask your child to copy you.
  - Clap three times, and have them copy.
  - Add foot tapping, marching in place, touching your nose, etc.

  Not recommended while driving!

Anticipating transitions, no matter how small, is a very proactive accommodation.

Tips for Problem Solving

Once you have a problem solving system in place, the journey to social independence begins in earnest. Even though I've told you not to go too fast, momentum is a good thing. Momentum moves forward on its own. Don't try to push it. When I ask you to slow down the moment, I'm really asking you to slow down the rush toward a neurotypical way of doing things. This will actually speed up the process of connecting with your child, and problem solving will move into high gear.

Let's wrap up this chapter with some tips for problem solving.

Be responsive, not reactive. Children do not participate well in a problem solving session if a parent is angry, judgmental, or shows intense emotions. That is a reactive, knee-jerk pattern that is so very easy to fall into when you are frustrated. Take a breath and calm yourself. It helps to know your intention. Listen and respond in a thoughtful and considered fashion. This is not always easy, but it's very important to strive for an emotional demeanor that is inviting for your child.

When you put your attention on a new way of responding, it can slow down the moment and bring the measure of calm you need.

Be patient and sensitive. See yourself as a confusion detective as you uncover the true nature of the problem. Switch from neurotypical thinking to Autistic thinking.

Maximize mutual understanding. Reciprocal communication is the key. You and your child need to understand each other, or you'll be working on two different problems. It's so important to build a rich set of well-tested accommodations. Literal language, comments before questions, and use of problem scales are just a few of the accommodations that come into play.

Minimize lecture. The number one problem I see is parents giving too much information too quickly. Yes, parents will need to take the lead in problem solving. Yes, you will initiate many of the interactions. That does not give you license to deliver a lecture. There is no quicker way to destroy your lines of communication. Minimize lectures to keep the momentum going.

Provide a space and a place for problem solving. Leave plenty of time in your schedule for children who are interested in tackling a problem. I recommend a space in the schedule and place in the home, even for short problem-solving "meetings." A physical problem jar is a great focal point for such a space and place.

* * *

Problem solving is more than problem solving. It is a social interaction. It helps build trust. It models a process your child can learn to use independently. It's a foundational element for socialization and authentic relationships.

17

Social Readiness

When is a child ready to move beyond the Preparation part of The Connection Formula and transition into the Socialization phase? If you have been interacting with your child, sharing social information with your child, problem solving with your child, then you have been socializing with your child.

When a parent asks about readiness for socialization, they are generally talking about their child's ability to socialize with other kids. They want to know: *When can my child go out and play? When will she be accepted by other children? When will he connect with the kids at the playground?*

In this part of the book we have raised big questions of *when* pertaining to a child's conceptual and emotional readiness. What about these day-to-day questions? It's not as if we can reach a given milestone on any kind of schedule, so the best question for any moment is: *what is my child's next step?*

No parent gets to raise their child in a single day. From time to time all need to consider their child's next step. For parents of an Autistic child, it's as if you get to watch the steps of social development under a microscope. Neurotypical children learn from play. They self-observe, self-correct, and then apply what they learn to new social situations. A child on the autism spectrum will be challenged in these areas. They need lots of preparation, and the work doesn't stop on the day they make a friend or have their first play date. You need to provide help at a very minute level. Like all parenting, it's a day-by-day process.

Here are a few questions to help assess your child's social readiness. We are looking for signs of social independence.

- ☐ Does my child have the tools to independently navigate problems and conflicts?
- ☐ Does my child have the resiliency to deal with new and unexpected social situations?
- ☐ Can my child accurately express their point of view?
- ☐ Is my child able to ask for help when it's needed?
- ☐ Does my child initiate problem solving, e.g. by independently using the problem jar?

These are all aspects of self-advocacy, an important part of social independence. In this chapter I'll elaborate on the idea of self-advocacy with the story of Ethan, a seventeen-year-old on the autism spectrum who found himself in a frustrating emotional paradox as he struggled to identify and articulate his point of view. It illustrates what I mean by social readiness with a view through that developmental microscope.

This is a complex little scenario that touches on many of the principles we have covered. And if it sounds complex to you, imagine how it felt to Ethan.

The Paradox Problem

Ethan's mother explained the situation this way: "We were planning a party for Saturday and had bought some shrimp cocktail to serve as an appetizer. The night before, Ethan's younger cousin visited. Ethan showed her the shrimp and basically let her eat most of it. The next day at the party, when we found out that most of the shrimp was gone, Ethan was very rude about the whole incident. He told us that we only got the shrimp because it was his favorite treat and so why should it matter if he let his cousin eat them."

She went on to say that Ethan was so angry and distraught when the whole thing came to light that he left the party to take a long walk. Truth be told, telling the story there in my office, the mother seemed more than a little upset herself. There always seems to be plenty of frustration to go around.

I was left to speak with Ethan alone. In order to make a discussion of the topic accessible to him I needed to break down the information – the facts of the incident (which were very much as his mother related) versus the heart of the incident (how Ethan thought and felt about it). Such discussions, of course, are a part of socialization. Socializing is not just for parties or playing games – it's involved in every human interaction, including the discussion I was about to have with Ethan. My main goal – by now I don't really need to repeat it – was to help him feel safe and understood.

Ethan at first repeated to me what he'd told his Mom. Why should she be concerned when he had equal rights to the family refrigerator? The shrimp had been chosen as an appetizer because it was his suggestion in the first place, so why couldn't he give them to his cousin? Frankly, it was a rather flimsy argument, yet he was sincerely trying to advocate for himself, and I was sincerely looking for a way to side with him – or, I should say, to *connect* with him and his emotional reality. Though he trusted me, he nonetheless grew agitated as we explored different views on whether he really had the right to give away the appetizer. The breakthrough came when he blurted out something close to the heart of his experience:

"I tried to avoid the problem!"

Here was the access ramp, his true point of view. He didn't really believe his own "right to the shrimp" argument, but it was all he'd been able to come up with to avoid the conflict. Avoiding conflict was important to Ethan, and as you'll see, that's what got him into the situation in the first place.

I needed to validate his point of view before we went any further. Remember: validate first.

"Oh," I said, as if a light bulb had just lit up over my head. "You saw the problem coming and you didn't want it to happen!"

"Yes!" he replied.

Now Ethan and I had our access ramp. (He, too, was working hard to find it; a sign of his emerging self-advocacy skills.) Here's the story that came out:

Ethan likes his younger cousin, and when she visited he cheerfully showed off the shrimp in the refrigerator. Well, the cousin likes shrimp too, and even knowing it was wrong, Ethan was powerless to stop her from helping herself. He avoided a conflict by letting her eat her fill. He didn't know how to speak up to her.

The next day, as luck would have it, Ethan was asked to fetch the shrimp and bring it to the guests. The appetizer was his idea, after all, so he was given the honor of serving it. As you can imagine, this was a very awkward moment for the young man, since he knew the "crime" would now be discovered – and he would be the one to deliver the evidence, quite literally, on a platter. He felt responsible as a witness and also because he had shown the shrimp to his cousin in the first place. So he hesitated. Again, he was just trying to avoid a conflict.

His reluctance to serve the shrimp was interpreted as selfishness and stubbornness. Under pressure, he eventually fetched the plate, hastily confessing in advance that "a lot of it is gone." Suddenly Ethan was in the center of a storm – exactly what he wished to avoid – as the interrogation and scolding began. The cousin's involvement quickly came to light, but she was not present, so Ethan took the brunt of the adults' irritation. *How could you let your cousin do that? She's younger than you, you should know better. Don't you know that was reserved for the party? Don't you know that costs money?*

And in this situation, it was impossible for Ethan to explain his point of view. Where a neurotypical kid might have said, "Hey, what do you want me to do, I can't control her!" – Ethan was left to struggle with conflicted feelings over his favorite cousin, his favorite snack, and his sense of right and wrong. For me this was the moment of revelation, when I saw the conflict from Ethan's point of view.

"Oh," I said as all of this came out. "Did anyone ever tell you about paradoxes? You wanted your cousin to enjoy the shrimp, but you also wanted to save it for the party." It was indeed a paradox – a word Ethan knew quite well – but it never occurred to him that such a thing could apply to his own emotions. It became a breakthrough moment for Ethan as he realized that it's possible – even normal – to have conflicting feelings at the same time. He was so amazed by this new insight that his agitation subsided immediately.

Do you see Ethan's point of view? I hope so. His family now does. And Ethan himself has better access to his own feelings, at least regarding this particular incident.

Since Ethan experienced the revelation that conflicting feelings are possible, he is better prepared to interact with his cousin. And because the adults around him understand the situation, he knows he has trusted coaches who will support him when tricky situations come up. In his relationship with his cousin, he has progressed into the Socialization phase of The Connection Formula. He has recognized that she is younger and less mature than he is – a huge step – and he is not so inclined to bow to her every whim. He has learned to seek the support of adults when it comes to managing conflicts with her, all because the adults now take the time to see things from his point of view. They make a conscious effort to nurture his self-advocacy skills.

Does this translate into better conflict management with people other than his cousin or scenarios not involving party appetizers? Perhaps. Having this one success to build on can only help when new situations arise. The "shrimp cocktail paradox" is a new feeling phrase, a new reference point, a step toward social independence.

* * *

Have another look at the checklist at the start of this chapter. Could we have checked any of those boxes for Ethan before this experience? Perhaps not. How about at the end? I would say yes, some progress was made.

Now consider your own child. You have the building blocks to bring things forward. The next part of the book will put them to use. We will focus on creating shared moments, implementing Family Fun Time, and then move on to play dates and beyond.

Part 3: Socialization

Creating Shared Moments

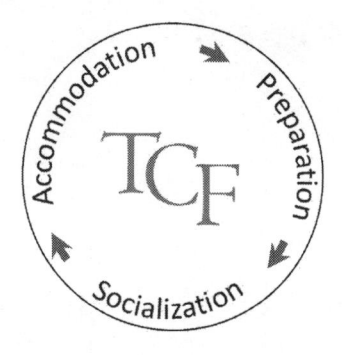

The feeling of being connected happens in what I call shared moments. Shared moments are what make the love visible.

18

Shared Moments

I believe children on the autism spectrum truly want to connect with others. I believe they want to feel connected to friends, family, and the community. Who really wants to feel all alone and disconnected from the world? No man is an island, after all. English poet John Donne wrote this almost four hundred years ago. When I was in Junior High chorus (not nearly as long ago!), I used to sing the song *People*, popularized by Barbara Streisand. I still remember the words: "People who need people are the luckiest people in the world..." I believed it then and believe it to this day. These words speak about the connections we feel with others. This feeling of being connected happens in what I call *shared moments*.

Having a meal with a friend is a shared moment; it's more about the friend than the food. I certainly have favorite restaurants, but I wouldn't trade my friends for even the best meal ever made! We instinctively feel that spending time with family and friends improves the quality of our lives, and so it does. The power of these shared moments has an almost sacred feeling. Imagine a dad playing catch with his son; a family baking cookies together; your best friend's wedding. Shared moments build and maintain relationships. Therefore we value these shared moments, whether large or small. We see their worth. Imagine the potential of a first date, the feeling you had seeing your newborn for the first time, or playing peek-a-boo with a toddler.

Shared moments are what make the love visible.

Now imagine that even though you want to have that feeling of connection, you do not see the value of shared moments. Let's back up even further – what if you don't see or feel the shared moment at all? You are simply unaware of it. Still, you crave the connection. Imagine you don't see how these "shared moments" will lead you there.

Adding to the confusion, people try to force you to have these moments by telling you to make eye contact, say hello to a neighbor, give grandma a hug – and you have no idea why. Think of it as a sort of color blindness; no amount of prodding is going to make you see the hidden colors. You simply don't perceive the value of these things, because for you they are not shared moments. They feel like dead-ends and a waste of time, not the building blocks of human interaction; not the gateway to the connections you long for.

Where does that leave us? What would motivate you to participate in these so-called shared moments if you simply couldn't perceive them? Think about this for a moment, and then turn the question back toward your child. What will motivate *them*?

We need to prove the value of a shared moment.

Proving the Value of the Moment

Proving the value of a shared moment – what could this possibly entail? If you try to force your idea of a shared moment on a child, you will often find yourself on an uphill journey that leads to frustration all around. Here you are, trying to figure out how to prove to your child that the things *you* recognize as shared moments are worth pursuing because they will help your child connect with others. All the while, what if your child is trying to do the same thing? What if your child is already trying to create shared moments with you and you are, in a sense, color blind to their attempts?

I have found that this is often the case. Some parents are no more able to accept their child's idea of a shared moment than the child is able to accept the parent's viewpoint. Something has to give in this standoff, and frankly, it has to be you, the parent. In due course it comes down to determining what is fun for your child, then finding a way to join with them.

Start by really listening carefully to your child's interests. Parent's say: "But they already talk too much about that TV show." Or: "I don't want to hear any more about all the variations of starfish in the world."

In other words: *Do I need to fake interest? It's boring to me!*

Well, when a child hands me a key to connect with them, I treasure it. I would not think of discarding it. It doesn't matter what their interest is. Remember, discussions of starfish and TV shows are not your end result. These are the means to an end. By engaging with your child, you're actually comforting them. You're learning to understand them, helping them feel safe. You may not be interested in the topic, but I *know* you're interested in what makes your child happy. What we're doing here is building a foundation so you can be more a part of their conversations and interactions. We are looking for shared moments. Let's not be fussy.

We're building a communication bridge to help a child socialize. We want *them* to want *us* to be part of the conversation. The goal is for the child to look forward to talking to us, to be eager to interact, and have fun interacting. That's the essence of a shared moment.

It's not so hard to prove the value of the moment when it's a moment your child already values.

Yielding Your End of the Moment

People connect by talking about everyday events. We may call it small talk, yet its value in creating shared moments is anything but small. However, some on the spectrum might not feel it as a shared moment. For one who does not feel the connection, small talk does not seem like a rational way to spend time. They might say we are wasting time talking, or feel stuck waiting for something of value to occur. Meanwhile, their head may be full of potential connection points that do have value to them. This is where it helps to yield your end of the shared moment. How? When your child offers a connection point, connect to it! Make connecting comments such as these:

👍 *You have interesting information about old-time baseball players.*

👍 *You know much more about computer games than I do.*

👍 *You know many facts about the state capitals.*

The Connection Formula

These give you a foot in the door, and make conversation valuable from your child's point of view. Then you build. Make related comments:

👍 *I saw a documentary about baseball history on TV once.*

👍 *You probably never heard of the first computer game I played.*

👍 *I learned about state capitals in fourth grade, and I have lived in five different states.*

Make your interests intersect for mutual benefit. Both of you can enjoy a conversation. This is the basis for many of the accommodations in the first part of the book, especially the ideas for keeping the conversation going, presented in Chapter 6. Now we are using accommodations to bring things forward. They become building blocks for authentic connections.

The Friendship Experience

Shared moments. Authentic connections. Social relatedness. What do these things really mean?

James is a very warm individual who likes to connect with others, although as a teenager on the autism spectrum, his idea of connection does not match up with neurotypical expectations. On the surface, it doesn't seem to be causing problems for him. He has lots of acquaintances. People are drawn to his outgoing personality. For a long time James himself did not see a problem. But he has no close friends.

How does James connect with others? For him, "connecting" means sharing a burst of information that interests him, after which he often walks away from the interaction.

"Hey James," you might say, "I hear you know all the state capitals. You must get good grades in geography." It's a conversation starter, and James responds in his own special way. "I like history better because I am learning about the industrial revolution which began in Britain in 1760." And off he goes, satisfied with the "conversation."

Perhaps this is one reason why James has many acquaintances but no deeper friendships. It's a stumbling block because James has not yet developed the perception necessary to navigate relationships with closer bonds. When we get closer to each other, the skills needed for an acquaintance relationship are not sufficient. Expectations change. We are expected to listen more intently, offer support, participate in longer conversations, mend hurt feelings, negotiate differences—just to name a few. There are social skills involved in all of this, yet skills alone are superficial when one does not perceive the nature of the shared moment. In other words, you can develop the skill to *appear* interested in what another person is saying, but it is no substitute for the ability to be genuinely interested in other people and their thoughts and ideas.

James does not realize he is substituting acquaintance skills for friendships, and he might believe that these acquaintances are his friends. Maybe some of his acquaintances will try to develop a friendship with him, and he might come to realize that more attention to the potential friend is necessary. Unfortunately, he might also accidently stop a friendship from blossoming. The longer James goes without having a friendship experience, the more catching up he will have to do. If he doesn't recognize how he appears from a neurotypical perspective, he could face frustrations in adulthood.

On the positive side, there are shared moments all over the place for him. We just have to keep throwing him a lifeline. When I interact with James, I yield my end of the moment in order to give him a sense of connection, if only for a few minutes longer. I ask specific questions about his interests in order to keep the conversation going. "Oh, I see you know about the industrial revolution. What were some of the changes that happened?" A conversation might be 99% about him and his interests and 1% about me. It's still a shared moment. He may gradually recognize that the conversation has value for both of us. At the very least, he finds that he is not having a negative experience. I do not try to pull him out of his comfort zone all at once. I let him enjoy himself.

When you yield the shared moment with a person like James, you become somebody they can connect with. When trust builds, you can move things forward with the social information they need.

James can take some feedback, but I do not call him out on every social misstep. I do not try to make him appear un-Autistic or give him a personality transplant. He has a big personality and will always be delightfully different. Still, he wants true friends and needs to know what that entails. Offer feedback gently and directly in just enough places, and it will reach critical mass.

"James, did you notice that person wanted to keep talking to you?"

"Oh, I need to think about other people more."

That is a big insight – a concept gap revealed. James is learning to self-observe.

What Is Social Relatedness?

Autistic children might not relate to shared moments as you do; this does not mean they can't experience one. James experiences shared moments all the time, but misses out on true friendships because the shared moments are not reciprocal. This can be very subtle.

Pay attention to your interactions with family, friends, acquaintances, and (especially) strangers. Notice how the quality of a shared moment depends on the nature of the relationship. What gives you this sense? The waitresses at a nearby restaurant are very friendly to me, but this does not mean they see me as their close friend. The subtle quality of our shared moments is understood. James is an extrovert, friendly to all, yet he might talk to his mom in the same way he talks to the clerk at a store. How will James come to perceive all the subtlety involved in the texture of his relationships, especially if those who try to help him never really stop to think about it themselves? We need to understand what makes a true shared moment tick.

It is social relatedness.

Adults offer all kinds of social instruction to Autistic children, but their words are premised on an innate understanding that is not mutual. To a child on the spectrum, anything that does not seem relevant is simply disregarded; the child's neurological makeup filters it out. So we need to make the information relevant. Yes, you can reinforce desired behaviors. However, getting a child to act the part doesn't make it real. My goal is always to provide *genuine* shared moments. We have to provide guidance that a child can conceptually relate to, and we have to do it in a way that feels emotionally safe.

That's what is involved in proving the value of a shared moment. It's a tall order, in part due to misconceptions about social relatedness. No, not just a child's misconceptions. There are many *neurotypical* misconceptions, the biggest of which is this: mistaking social manners for true social relatedness.

> **Social Manners and Social Relatedness Are Not the Same**
>
> I once attended a conference on autism where an audience member – a gentleman on the autism spectrum – expressed disappointment at his failure to make friends. He had heard that friends often exchange greeting cards, so he sent holiday cards to everyone he knew in order to start some friendships. No one sent a card in return. The man was upset and confused.
>
> Should his approach have worked?
>
> The recipients were not his friends to begin with, so it it's not surprising that none of them responded. This fellow's emotional pain at the perceived rejection was palpable in the room.
>
> I wish I could have handed him the key to social connection right then and there, but there is no instant answer. A long process is involved, a process of building self-esteem, gaining confidence, and nurturing small successes. There is no overnight solution, but there is always hope. It's a journey, not a race. Even if autism could be instantly "cured," how would this restore a lifetime of missed social experience? How does one go back and acquire all the essential social learning of childhood? Just think of the countless social interactions we take for granted, but that he had lacked for his entire life. What is involved in acquiring all those missing interactions and the emotional connectedness that comes with them?
>
> This is the difficulty with social manners: they do not create social connections in and of themselves. Simply put, you have to live it.

So what is social relatedness? Let's talk first about what it's not. I often hear people talk about socializing in terms of social manners and social rules. Social rules and manners include such things as taking turns, saying thank you, offering your guest something to drink, waiting your turn in line, not interrupting when someone is talking...the rules of etiquette fill advice columns, blogs, and volumes of books. Notice how much learned behavior is involved. Why do we follow these conventions? What is their purpose? On the surface it is to be polite and not make any social missteps. Looking a bit deeper, there is a widespread view that people will judge your character based on your grasp of social etiquette, which is all too true. I will certainly not argue with the importance of social manners. Clearly society expects these skills in all of us. Doors of opportunity may open or close based on one's social manners. Indeed, the skills are needed if one expects to fit in and thrive in the world.

But are social manners a substitute for social relatedness? Do polished social skills mean that you understand how to connect with someone else? Does proper table etiquette help you feel safe and understood? Does remembering to say "please" and "thank you" have anything to do with relating to another person's point of view? Do good manners mean you are connected to your family and the community? That you have true friends? That you feel loved?

No, of course not. Not at all.

Think of James. He's an extrovert. He'll look you in the eye and shake your hand and call you by name. As far as manners are concerned, he does a lot of things just right. He's trying hard to follow all the rules that have been given to him. Yet he has still not reached his potential for authentic connections.

Socializing means connecting with other people – truly connecting, on an innate level that most of us do not even need to think about. Real social relatedness is reciprocal. Both parties share a mutual understanding in a mutually understood world. This capability to have an authentic, meaningful connection with others is exactly what is impacted by autism.

Parents are understandably concerned that their child will have a hard life without the necessary social skills. With or without these skills, a child will have a much harder life without true social relatedness. Some professionals focus on social manners; their work is very important, and can be extremely helpful. True social relatedness, however, is something of a different sort. I am focused on this aspect of socialization. It is, I believe, no less than the key to happiness.

Shared Moments

The key to happiness? Really? Well, how happy can you be if you don't understand the people in your life – and they don't understand you? This is what I work on with the children that I see.

When I first meet with a child at my office, we discuss why they have come. Sometimes these children have skills in areas that totally elude me – they may be good spellers, for example, or have a keen interest in math or history or geography, subjects that I readily admit I do not excel in. Still, I yield my end of the moment to the child's interests, and eventually this gives us a common frame of reference and allows us to connect. To be honest, many of these children initially wonder what I could possibly have to offer. "I'm very good at being happy," I tell them. "My job is to make sure kids are happy, and usually kids are happy when they have friends." I may not be good at those other things, I explain, but it's okay for us to be different.

And so the process of social relatedness begins, with shared moments like these.

19

Job Description for a Social Coach

So we have reached the Socialization part of The Connection Formula. What happens now? It's not as if there's a well-drawn boundary for new territory with new rules. You use the tools you have been learning all along. Now, though, you get a job title: you become your child's social coach.

The way you do this job is flexible because it has to be. Every child is different, every parent is different. However, certain qualities are uncompromising if you are going to be effective. The next chapter will put you to work. First let's review some job requirements.

A social coach does not jump to socialization too soon. Don't try to teach socialization before you can accurately communicate with your child. Use accommodations to build the groundwork. Implement just one new accommodation at a time, and then add more as you and your child are comfortable. Above all, a child needs to feel safe and understood in order to thrive.

Do the necessary preparation. Socialization can't be taught before your child is conceptually and emotionally ready. Prioritize connection above correction. You cannot lead until your child is able to follow.

A social coach proves their worth to their child. As strange as it may sound for parents, you'll need to earn your child's trust. That is, you'll need to show the relevance of your social information by presenting it in a way that is accessible and meaningful. When parents try to teach socialization in a neurotypical manner, they confuse their child and lose credibility. Prove that socialization is worth the effort.

The Connection Formula

A social coach does not look at autism through neurotypical glasses. Many think that interventions designed for neurotypical children will be just as successful for children on the autism spectrum. They won't be. This is looking at autism through a neurotypical lens: *My child yells because he has autism. We must teach him to stop yelling.*

Don't make that mistake.

A good social coach views things quite differently: *My child is yelling because that is an appropriate response to the situation* as he perceives it. *We need to understand his experience and get to the bottom of this yelling.*

The difference is HUGE!!!

A social coach is willing to step out of their comfort zone. Many parents try to work from within their own comfort zone, where the child is expected to make all the difficult changes. Unfortunately this approach is often encouraged by the professionals around them. Then, when the system fails the child, parents believe it is their child who has failed.

There's work to be done by both child and coach; a good social coach learns how to facilitate the process.

A social coach explores a different way of teaching. Teaching socialization to Autistic children is quite different from teaching it to neurotypical children. Some parents believe that forcing their child to be around other kids will make them happier. I use this analogy: if your child has a reading disability, will leaving them in a room full of books help them to read? Without the specific help they need, you will only stress them out. Autism is a social learning disability. The last thing you want to do is add stress and anxiety.

Negative socialization experiences leave lasting wounds. Some people are overly eager and push Autistic children into socializing too quickly. They are impatient to move forward and don't see why I have certain guidelines that only seem to slow things down. Well, that's the whole point. I am *trying* to slow things down...to a pace that the child can tolerate.

Let's say that Zachery has no friends. Concerned, his mom devises a plan to help him socialize. She is aware of a children's party down the street that her friend is hosting for some nieces and nephews. Zach has been to this neighbor's house before, but never when other children were present. Knowing that Zach would refuse to go to a party, Mom does not tell him about it. As far as Zach knows, it will be a routine visit where he gets to play his electronic game while his mom and her friend chat over coffee nearby. So Zach walks into the house with his mom, and finds himself in a room full of other kids.

Mom envisions that Zach will find a way to participate in the fun. But he is on the autism spectrum. How do you think this all works out?

I have heard many stories along these lines, and let me tell you they do not end well. From a child's point of view, such an incident can be perceived as a profound violation of trust, and the emotional wound can last a very long time. Some children manage to hold it together outwardly, but the wound is still there. If they're able to express their feelings, they report that they felt tricked or betrayed. Others might run from the room. In the worst case, a meltdown ensues – all the more humiliating if it occurs in front of the other children. I know teenagers whose social anxiety can be traced back to bad experiences they had at age five, six, or seven. A negative social experience will discourage a child from ever wanting to try again.

Do not try to trick an Autistic child into socializing. The "sink or swim" approach is just too risky. Even if a child is told about the event beforehand, forced socialization can be a traumatic experience. In a way you're lucky if your child becomes emotional because at least you will know about the wound. A strong emotional reaction might be their best defense mechanism, an obvious signal of distress. It will not be convenient, but at least you'll have an idea of what they're feeling. Other children will simply shut down, hiding their anxiety and masking the problem...for now.

So the stakes are high. How does one involve a child like Zach in socialization? Well that's the topic of this entire book. Once the accommodations and preparations are in place, you need to put all the pieces together and step up your game as a social coach.

A social coach gets to know their child's world. Creating reliable communication, identifying concept gaps, assessing a child's emotional readiness for social experiences – these are all skills that I teach to willing parents on their way to being social coaches. These skills require a shift of viewpoint that can be very difficult for some. Parents will watch me successfully interact with their child, or they will attend a workshop in which I offer specific insights and tools, and it will all click...for a moment. Permanent change, though, is elusive. All too often a switch is thrown and the parent clicks back into old routines. I know this switch well – I'm neurotypical, too, after all – and I have to keep flipping back to autism mode. It does get easier with practice. It is absolutely possible to autism-ize your thinking.

A social coach learns on the job. It's a job you didn't apply for, but somehow you got it anyway.

Will you embrace it?

20

Family Fun Time

A social coach learns to prove the value of a shared moment, and the most solid proof you can offer your child is the actual experience of shared moments. How do you do that? The best way I know is to have fun together.

The basic idea behind Family Fun Time is simple: Plan 20 or 30 minutes for structured games and fun activities with your child, involving other family members when practical. Do this with regularity – once a day or a few times a week, whatever your schedule allows.

That, on the surface, is all there is to it. Just try to be consistent. Once a week, every week, is better than a burst of ambition for a several days in a row followed by months with no structure.

Family Fun Time is a time when you water the seeds you have planted for connection, insight, and trust. It provides the opportunity to give guidance in the most socially accessible environment you can create for your child, and prepares the way for successful problem solving so that no one feels defeated.

The best part is this: you and your child get to enjoy spending time together while you learn what makes each other tick, all in a light-hearted way. That's the ideal model for Family Fun Time.

* * *

The details are best shown by example, so in this chapter we'll look in on a mom who has done a pretty good job of implementing Family Fun Time. Her eleven year old son, Jonathan, is on the autism spectrum. His older sister Kate is a neurotypical thirteen-year-old. They are all familiar with the activities and the accommodations, groundwork you should put in place well in advance. This family has done this before, and although not everything works out perfectly, Mom knows how to keep things moving and is ready with a backup plan at every turn.

This extended case study illustrates how the ingredients of The Connection Formula can be mixed together to create a safe and fun social training ground in your child's life. Things will almost certainly be different in your home, but the underlying principles still apply.

> **What If It Doesn't Work?**
>
> If you try too much too soon, then Family Fun Time won't work out very well. The good news is that you'll learn more about your child's needs. Cycle back and bring some appropriate accommodations into play. Review the Preparation part of the book and look at your child's conceptual and emotional readiness. If you work with the Family Fun Time model consistently, you will always be uncovering some new area to work on. There is always a next step, so count it as progress when you discover what it is.
>
> I know there's a lot to do here. Honestly, you might need to reach out to other parents to get support and share ideas. I'm presenting a big picture; it's okay to pick one small detail that you can work on.
>
> Don't try to take off from the end of the runway. Back up as far as necessary to make socialization accessible for your child.

The most important principle to keep in mind about this training ground: it has to be tilted to give your child a track record of success. Family Fun Time has to be fun! It is a microcosm full of interactions of the sort your child will encounter when socializing outside the home, but don't throw everything in there all at once. Manage it in a way that motivates your child to want more.

Setting Up the Idea

> *It's about 4:15pm. Family Fun Time begins at 4:30. Mom looks over at the schedule on the refrigerator and sees that Jonathan has put a "thumbs up" sticker next to the time slot.*

Family Fun Time

This is our first indication of how prepared this mom is. She has taken the time to consistently make a visual schedule for each day, and clearly Jonathan is familiar with it and fully engaged. The "thumbs up" symbol confirms that he looks forward to the activities.

This accommodation of a visual schedule is a great idea, even if your child is not as tuned into it as Jonathan. Some families use them only for especially busy days. Jonathan's mom has found that it comforts her son when he knows what to expect on a daily basis. She reviews the schedule with him at bedtime the night before, and as an added bonus she discovered he becomes more fully engaged when he can make his opinion known by using the "thumbs up" and "thumbs down" stickers that she found at a craft store.

Organizing the Environment

> *The clock is counting down, so Mom goes to the closet and pulls out the activities box. Inside are all the "fun time" items, including trivia cards, games, activity books, writing and drawing supplies, a timer – and some small whiteboards.*

One can never seem to have too many whiteboards. This mom will be using three of them. Of course paper, easels, and good old-fashioned blackboards are also an option.

An organized environment is very important. You will want as few distractions as possible. The structure of the environment is a way of showing expectations—it is time to stay in *this* area; it is time to do *this* activity. The environment itself sends strong social cues, so make sure it is clearly defined and sends the signals you want. This will be comforting to your child and easier for you.

The activities box is the key ingredient, but the room itself is just as important. Try to see the environment from your child's point of view as we zoom in on these important considerations:

> **The room** you use for Family Fun Time should have as few distractions as possible. In a perfect world you will have an area to store the games and toys you are *not* using so they can be kept out of sight. Too much visual stimuli can be confusing and

distracting. It is hard to know where to look. If your child is impulsive, then it will be very tempting for them to over-attend to the wrong game or toy. Organizing the environment is something I do out of respect for the child's social learning style. To do otherwise is asking too much of them too soon.

The play area should be well-defined within the room. When your child comes in, do they automatically know where to go? A small, nearly empty room with a door works very well, but not everyone will have this luxury. A large open-concept room will work if you arrange a smaller play area within the room. A small, cluttered room will require a bit more creativity to eliminate distractions and create a clearly defined play area. The play area may be obvious to you, but you might need to take things a step further to define it for your child. Ottomans lined up in row with an opening for walking through is a nice option. Or chairs can be lined up so that their backs define the play area. The goal is not to hold your child prisoner; it is to define the space so they will know what to attend to.

Think in terms of a playing surface such as a table or a cleared space on the floor. If you use the floor, colored floor mats work nicely to define the play surface. Another alternative is to use painter's tape to delineate the playing surface.

I keep the environment organized even for a child who doesn't seem distracted by extra items. A sparse environment can feel calming, relaxing, and safe. Certainly you can experiment if your child is truly enjoying Family Fun Time. When and if you make changes to the play area, please consider letting your child know why. When neurotypical people make changes and don't explain why, we can actually appear irrational to someone on the autism spectrum. Since you want your child to trust you in the social-emotional world – as I'm sure you do – then don't risk looking too illogical. That might decrease their trust in you – exactly the opposite of our goal.

The activities box is the final element in our organized environment. Family Fun Time is not the time to be running around the house looking for things. Have all the activities ready to go before you start. You'll want easy access to what you need, when you need it. Having the activities in a box or storage container is very helpful. The box should be positioned such that you are clearly the one managing it. Keep it behind you if the space allows. The purpose is to minimize distractions and send clear social cues.

Organizing the Schedule

> Mom looks in the activities box for her notes on today's agenda.

Yes, she keeps notes. They help her stay organized and keep promises. Promises are important to Jonathan. His mom is building trust.

> First up is Hangman. Mom sees that it's Kate's turn to lead the game and the theme is movie titles, so she puts this at the top of the activities list on a whiteboard. Her notes remind her that she promised a game of Apples to Apples, so Mom adds it to the list.
>
> Movie trivia is the final activity, so it goes onto the list as #3. An important fourth item completes the schedule:
>
> #1. Hangman: Movie titles (Kate leads).
> #2. Apples to Apples (3 rounds).
> #3. Movie trivia
> #4. Stop

You may be wondering, "Do you *really* want me to use schedules and timers for Family Fun Time?" Yes, I do!

Schedules provide a calming structure for children on the spectrum. Structure requires planning, and time to plan is exactly what you don't have when things are getting busy. Establish a structure in advance. It is easy to relax it later if things are going smoothly, but nearly impossible to create structure in the moment when all is in chaos.

It is important to familiarize your child with the use of schedules and timers prior to the first Family Fun Time. As with other accommodations, don't try to introduce this at the last minute. You should make your child aware that there is a schedule, but you don't need to make a big deal out of it. Review the information about schedules in Chapter 10 for thoughts on how to introduce the idea.

> *With the schedule complete, Mom takes out the timer from the activities box and places it where everyone will be able to see it.*

A schedule won't mean much to your child if they cannot perceive the structure it creates. I like to use a large Time Timer® because it makes it easy for the whole family to see how much time is left. This is not just about finishing on time, nor is it solely about teaching and reinforcing the idea of structure and schedules. Our purpose here is not to teach your child to follow a schedule. Our purpose is to *ground the activities in our neurotypical reality so they do not seem like random events*. In other words, make life predictable. There is no need for a big lecture. The best way to do this is by demonstration. Just keep things moving, direct your child's attention to the timer now and then, and yes, do try to finish on time. (That is a goal for you, not your child.)

Beginning-Middle-End

"Okay," you might think. "I'll go along with this schedule idea, but why is 'Stop' listed on the schedule? Obviously we'll stop when we reach the end."

Well remember, the concept of *beginning-middle-end* is not obvious to all children. Transitions can be very difficult for some. Item #4 on the list is actually quite important because it shows a definite stopping point for the activities. Do all you can to make expectations clear.

Preparing the Activities

> *On a second whiteboard Mom writes out the alphabet. This will be used as a reference in the letter-guessing game of Hangman. It's an accommodation for Jonathan, who finds it easier to keep track of which letters have been guessed when he can see the whole alphabet written out.*
>
> *Mom places a third small whiteboard on the table—this one will be used to play the game. Leaving nothing to chance, she*

> writes the order of play at the top of this board:
> Kate
> Jonathan
> Mom
> The Apples to Apples game is across the room on a bookshelf, so Mom fetches it and adds it to the activities box, where it will be instantly available when needed and not be a distraction in the meantime.

Smooth transitions are very important as you manage the supplies. When you take the next activity from the box, will your child stay engaged, or become distracted? Your own shift of focus is a social cue. How will your child read it?

I call these *micro-transitions*. Micro-transitions open the door to social missteps if they are not handled efficiently. For example, if there is even a small delay while readying the next activity (for example, if Mom has to go find the Apples to Apples game), a child might think that the activities are over and get up to leave. Then, if corrected, they might feel self-conscious or confused. So much for the fun.

Micro-transitions, then, are tiny waiting moments that need to be filled. With Jonathan, quick transitions work best. With other children, a running commentary might work if the transition takes longer:

👍 *I'm taking the next activity from the box...And here it is!*

It takes a bit of trial and error to figure out what works best for a particular child. Make these micro-transitions as fast and seamless as possible, and fill the time with running commentary as needed.

> Mom inspects the activity books which she keeps in the box. She makes sure that there are still plenty of available activities, and puts a bookmark on a movie-related picture-find puzzle page in case it will be needed.

What are the activity books for? They are not on the agenda. As we'll see, these are waiting activities. If there is an unexpected delay (the doorbell, a phone call), then waiting activities will be needed to fill the gap. We will see some examples soon. This is one snag you can avoid by being aware of micro-transitions and "polishing your act" to manage them smoothly. It's your job to minimize all the variables that can go wrong. Even so, things *will* go wrong, and when they do, that becomes part of the program. You will learn the most effective accommodations for your child.

False Starts and Big Discoveries

> *Finally, Mom calls the kids to the family room. "Come on kids, it's Game Time!"*

No, she doesn't call it Family Fun Time. You can call it anything you want. *Art Time, Music Time, Puzzle Time, Tell Your Favorite Joke Time,* and even (of course!) *Family Fun Time.*

On her first attempts, she called it *Fun Time*. Things did not work out so well, and "fun time" got a bad reputation...so she rebranded it. What went wrong for our mom? A couple things. First, she had pulled Jonathan away from his favorite video game. "Stop playing your game, it's Fun Time!" Now *that* did not go over well. More on this soon.

Second, Jonathan was unable to tolerate waiting, and his mom was unprepared with waiting activities. When there was any delay between activities, Jonathan would become extremely frustrated. To her credit, Mom had stayed mostly calm, and fortunately she already had some tools in place. She brought out a 1-5 problem scale, and learned that waiting was indeed a BIG problem for Jonathan. Well, she already knew as much based on his frustration, but the problem scale at least calmed Jonathan down, so she turned it into a question game, asking him about waiting for dessert, waiting in movie lines, waiting for school vacation...anything she could think of. That's how she made an interesting discovery: Jonathan perceived *all* waiting in the same way, no matter how long or short. For some children on the spectrum, any sort of delay can feel like a deep loss, as if the hoped-for event will never happen. This concept gap is not uncommon.

As you can see, this mom managed to mine her "false start" for information, and gained an important insight about her son.

Family Fun Time helps uncover concept gaps. When these are

obstacles to your child's enjoyment of life, you need to find ways to uncover them, work around them, climb over them, and – if possible – remove them.

Don't expect to get things exactly right the first time.

Transitioning In

> *Jonathan arrives right away for game time.*

Mom has definitely learned from her first attempt when she pulled him away from his video game. Now she schedules game time as a break between chores and homework, which eases the transition. As I mentioned in the previous section, it wasn't always so easy. Even though he enjoys the activities, transitions are difficult for Jonathan. For one thing, he seems to find it hard to change his focus. But he does not mind changing focus from his chores!

Changing focus is only part of the problem with transitions. Another difficulty involves knowing what to expect from moment to moment. Springing some spontaneous fun may work well with some children, but Jonathan likes to know what's coming next. We have already seen Mom's solution to make transitions easier: the visual schedule which she keeps on the refrigerator and reviews with Jonathan each night. We know Jonathan is engaged with the visual schedule (he uses those "thumb's up/thumbs down" stickers), and often he arrives for game time without being called.

Keeping Things Moving

> *Jonathan arrives first, but older sister Kate is delayed because she is texting a friend. Uh-oh. Mom is well aware that any unexpected delays have an impact on her son. She is also well prepared, so she jumps right into a waiting activity. In this case it's a "Who in this family?" question game.*

So Fun Time hasn't even started and we already need a waiting activity. It goes like this: Mom thinks of a question about someone in the family and sees if Jonathan can guess who it is.

The Connection Formula

> *Mom starts the waiting activity by saying, "**Who in this family**..."*
> *– and pauses for suspense (the pause also lets her think of a question) –*
> *"...likes to see every movie at least 3 times in a row?"*
> *Jonathan has played this game before and says, "Me!"*
> *Mom teases him, "Are you sure it's not Dad?", and quickly adds, "That's a joke, by the way."*
> *Jonathan responds, "I know it's a joke, Dad always falls asleep during movies." Mom adds, "He might enjoy sleeping, but that is definitely not the same as enjoying the movie." Both Mom and Jonathan laugh.*

Meltdown averted, but Mom still has to keep things moving...

Making Everything Fun

> *At this moment Kate comes to the table. Without missing a beat Mom gets things underway. "Kate it's your turn to lead Hangman and the topic is movie titles."*
> *Kate draws the Hangman diagram on a whiteboard while trying to think of a movie title. This is another wait for Jonathan, so Mom asks, "Who in this family...likes to text the most?"*
> *Jonathan answers, "Kate!"*
> *Kate responds, "Hey! I'm trying to think!"*
> *Mom replies, "Okay, we'll be quiet for 30 seconds." And she mimes that her lips are sealed by a zipper. Jonathan sees this as part of the fun and plays along by being quiet, too*

This mom is really on her toes. She is well-practiced at using a question game to keep Jonathan's interest, and she knows how to give very specific instructions and make everything fun. Even when asking for quiet, she makes it fun by theatrically exaggerating her own efforts to stay silent. I find that exaggerated gestures are very effective at conveying social expectations in an accessible way, though this accommodation might not be for everyone.

In the past Jonathan's mom simply hushed him: *Be quiet, your sister is thinking.* That led to more than one meltdown. Now she knows she has to be "on" during Fun Time. It's a more high-energy approach up front, but it spares emotional backlash. This energy level can be very tiring at first, but it does get easier with practice. Plus, "fun tired" is much more enjoyable than "meltdown tired."

Letting It Be One-Sided

> *Finally Kate announces, "Okay, I have a movie in mind." Mom is once again mindful of Jonathan's attention as Kate takes time to mark the letter spaces on the whiteboard. This time Mom uses the movie picture-find puzzle from the activities box. She finds the page quickly. (Now you see why she used a bookmark.) And of course she provides a pencil.*
>
> *Jonathan knows the routine with the picture-find puzzle. He can choose to try to find one or two, or he can say, "No thanks." Without saying a word, he picks up the pencil and immediately finds one of the hidden items. Kate announces she is ready. Jonathan is looking for his second item.*

Now the others are waiting for Jonathan, but that's okay. Family Fun Time is allowed to be one-sided. By its nature, it is slanted toward the child on the autism spectrum. Yes, family dynamics can make this tricky at times. If sister Kate was not so patient with the process, things would be messier. Or she simply would be allowed to opt out. Bringing siblings on board is a huge topic which I do not have space to cover in this book. Obviously the process will vary greatly based on the age and needs of the children. If a sibling is just not able to handle the one-sided nature of the activities, do something special with them at another time. The same applies if more than one sibling is on the spectrum. Ideally everyone can participate together, but life is not always ideal.

Taking Turns

> *Jonathan locates a second picture-find item and now is ready. Mom points to the order-of-play on the agenda and tells him it's his turn to guess a letter.*

Pointing to the order-of-play is not just a random act. Mom is supporting communication with a visual accommodations.

> Jonathan looks at the board and guesses the letter "E". His sister fills it in:
>
> _ _ _ _ _ _ _ _   _ E _ _
>
> Mom crosses out the 'E' on the alphabet whiteboard:
>
> A B C D É F G H I J K L M
> N O P Q R S T U V W X Y
>
> She used to erase the letters, but has learned that crossing them out is the best way to help Jonathan to keep track of the already-guessed letters without confusing him.
>
> Mom then guesses, "I." Kate fills in two more letter positions:
>
> _ I _ _ I _ _   _ E _ _
>
> And suddenly Jonathan says "I know what it is!"
> Kate answers, "Wait until your turn... let Mom go first."

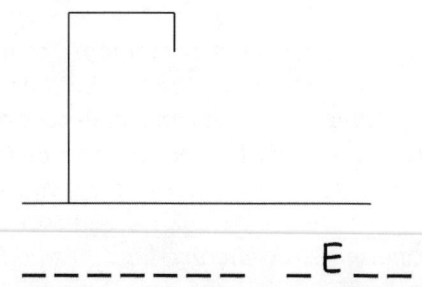

The concept of taking turns is difficult for Jonathan, as it is for many children on the spectrum. Going out of turn in this situation at home might not be a big deal, whereas socializing outside the home is a different story. It can be off-putting to peers and potential friends, so his mom has been looking for ways to give him social information about it.

She jumps at this opportunity.

> "You're very smart to get the answer so fast. The rules say it is my turn, so I will take ten seconds to think, and if I don't get the answer it will be your turn."

Notice that Mom does not give Jonathan a choice. True, much of The Connection Formula so far has been about accommodating Autistic children because that is the part most people skip. Still, we look for ways to lead. Accommodation isn't acquiescing; *connect before correct* doesn't mean we don't correct at all. We don't give up our leadership position; quite the contrary, we connect in order to *gain* a leadership position by becoming someone your child can understand and follow. That's the secret to being an effective social coach.

Mom wants to move things forward, and has confidence in her connection with Jonathan. Still, accommodations are needed. Now we see why she wrote the turn-taking order on the whiteboard. She points to it so her ruling will not seem arbitrary.

Winning and Losing

> To keep things fun, Mom makes a show of thinking about the answer. "I'm thinking...I'm thinking..."
>
> Her exaggerated befuddlement makes it clear to Jonathan that he will indeed get his turn.
>
> "I'm thinking..." she says. "And..."
>
> "...I have no idea. Your turn, Jonathan."
>
> Jonathan yells out, "Finding Nemo!"

I guess we'll never know if Jonathan's mom really knew the answer. (Did *you* know the answer?) If I was playing this game I would surely not have known the answer first, and if I knew the child well enough and thought they would get the joke, I would not hesitate to add a little teasing suspense. I use a good bit of over-acting when it is appropriate for the child.

On the other hand, if I did know the answer, I might go another way and take the opportunity to make a positive social interaction out of winning and losing:

The Connection Formula

👍 *I think I know the answer and you think you know the answer. The rules say it is my turn. Is it okay if I guess first?*

Much depends on the child's ability to handle winning and losing. If a child is sensitive to losing, I would possibly pretend I did not know the answer. In such cases it might be better to simply avoid win/lose games, at least initially. There are ways to work up to them. For example, I might say:

👍 *I will tell you my answer and you tell me if you think I'm right or wrong.*

Or you could both write your answers down and compare them. This gives your child a job to do, and may ease them into this type of game. Eventually you want your child to be comfortable with the rules they will encounter when outside the home.

Build In Success

If your child has trouble with losing, then begin with activities which minimize competition. Even the game of Bingo can be hard for some children; they can become frustrated if their number isn't called. There are Picture Bingo games designed so that every picture is on each card. In other words, everyone wins. It is a way to play Bingo while avoiding the stress of losing.

Other types of noncompetitive activities include: art, music, books, video clips, Mad Libs, puzzles, Legos, building blocks, joke time, interviews (questions planned in advance), and questionnaires (what's your favorite color, food, game, song, videogame, etc.). Look on educational web sites for other fun ideas.

Remember, Family Fun Time is a place to discover where your child needs guidance. And they need to feel safe and understood as you offer that guidance. Striking this balance takes some trial and error; try to err on the side of "safe and understood." Hold the intention of being a good social coach.

Make Encouraging Comments

> Jonathan seems quite enthusiastic about Finding Nemo. "It was made in 2003 and directed by Andrew Stanton..."
>
> Mom used to let Jonathan talk longer about his preferred interests during Fun Time. She has a great deal of patience and likes to see him happy. However, she realizes that other people will not be as patient; excessive talking about movies won't necessarily help him make friends. His sister gets tired of hearing about this topic, too.

Mom will gently redirect him. First, she gives him a compliment:

> "You have an amazing memory for movie trivia. I like the way your brain works!"

Always be sure to make encouraging comments. Sometimes, this is easier said than done. Some children find compliments strange and don't understand their purpose. If this is the case, then be sure you explain their purpose. (See *About Compliments* in Chapter 13.)

Mom's compliment at least got Jonathan's attention, so she goes on to redirect his focus away from his discussion of movie trivia. How? By connecting to his interest:

> "Movie trivia is #3 on the list, and there is time in the schedule for it." Again, she gives visual reinforcement by pointing to timer and the activities list.

Mom knows that Jonathan will need more direct information regarding too much talk about one topic and how it might bore other people. For now he is making progress connecting with the family on a growing variety of interests, and she doesn't want him to feel beat up from too many social instructions. She also notices that when she provides movie-themed activities, Jonathan seems more flexible and willing to investigate other interests. He is also getting better at listening to other family members. He just seems more relaxed.

The Autistic children I work with often come to me with a great deal of hidden stress. First, I use accommodations to help them feel safe and to help me understand them. I yield my end of the shared moment and allow the child to express their own interests. That lets me look for connecting logic. Next, I find a way to give them a footing in the neurotypical way of interacting. With these pieces in place, the child is more relaxed, the adults are more relaxed, and the shared moments begin to occur naturally.

Handling Criticism

> Mom gives Jonathan some concrete choices: "Would you like to erase the Hangman whiteboards, continue working on the picture-find, or something else?"
>
> Jonathan says in a firm tone of voice, "Mom you said white boardzzzz," exaggerating the plural s sound.
>
> What on earth could he mean? Mom realizes that for Jonathan there is technically only one hangman board – the one with the hangman picture on it. The alphabet is on a different whiteboard. Still, his tone sounds more than a little rude.

How does Mom handle criticism from her son? In the past she was exasperated by his literal critiques, but she has figured out that the literal structure of things keeps him emotionally grounded, and that no rudeness was intended. This awareness helps her reprogram her response.

> In a calm and kind tone of voice, Mom says, "You are right! There is only one whiteboard with the hangman picture on it. The other whiteboard just has the alphabet. I'm sorry I wasn't clear. Would you like to erase both the hangman board and the alphabet board?"

To help him do well in broader social circles, she will need to teach him about the concept of rudeness and make him aware of how he is viewed by others. At the moment her best judgment tells her he is not emotionally ready for this more advanced concept.

> Jonathan takes Mom's response in stride and erases both boards.

Family Fun Time

Handling Interruptions

> The next activity is Apples to Apples, but Mom's cell phone rings just as Kate starts to deal the cards. It's Dad and she has missed a previous call from him. During Fun Time there is a "No cell phones" policy.
>
> Mom says, "Kate and Jonathan, I need your help. I know this is a no cell phone time, but I have missed two calls from your dad and think I should answer. Is breaking the no cell phone rule a small, medium, or big problem?"
>
> Kate answers first and says, "It is a very small problem."
>
> Jonathan chimes in, "It is a negative ten problem!"
>
> Mom knows this means it is not a problem at all.

The problem-scale vocabulary has taken hold in this family, and it has proven very helpful. There is little guessing about Jonathan's feelings when he expresses them this way.

> Once again, a waiting activity is required. Mom brings out a second picture and gives both of her children the challenge of finding five hidden items. (She is very specific with numbers.) The kids study the puzzle. On the phone Mom explains that it is "GT" (Game Time). Dad knows the no cell phone rule and ends the call quickly.

It has been a long time coming: both children are able to interact independently as they look at the puzzle together. It may not seem like much to other parents, but this mom is thrilled to see potential for even more successful social family moments.

Structure Before Spontaneity

Can things really go this smoothly? Yes, it is possible. To get here, you may need to establish a number of accommodations in advance and uncover a lot of concept gaps. And you need detailed planning, as our mom is demonstrating in this scenario. Yes, spontaneity is allowed during Family Fun Time – and even encouraged. But as I've mentioned, it's better to have too much structure than not enough. Structure will not arise in the

The Connection Formula

> moment without some advance planning. Even little details – like having a pencil at hand when it's needed – are very important for keeping Fun Time running smoothly.
>
> Also keep in mind that our scenario assumes a family with several months of experience, and it has not been without its challenges. Don't feel badly about making mistakes, because this is certainly a process of trial and error.
>
> It's important to plan as many specifics as possible to create and maintain the structure of an activity. As our scenario proceeds to the game of Apples to Apples, you'll see that Mom has learned to break down each aspect of the game into smaller steps so she can carefully watch the details.

Watching and Guiding

For those who are not familiar with Apples to Apples, I should explain that it's a popular word game. In each round, one player serves as the judge of the most "creative, humorous or interesting" word match which the other players choose from cards that they are dealt. Judging is subjective, and as a result the game involves a great deal of social interaction. Doubtless this is one reason why it is so popular.

There are many possible variations on the rules. A full game might last for more than half an hour, but Jonathan would not be able to sustain his attention that long, so the family generally plays three rounds, and everyone gets to be a judge. Remember that "3 rounds" was included on the activities whiteboard. This may seem like a small detail, but it sets the appropriate expectations ahead of time. Certain details can be incredibly important, but it varies greatly from child to child. This mom has learned that things go more smoothly for her son when the turn-taking and game-length details are written down in advance. For now he depends on this predictable structure.

> Kate has dealt the cards, and Mom says, "Kate, you are the first person to judge." This means Kate must draw a green card and read it aloud for the others to match.

Kate already knows that she is the judge. Mom is making things clear for Jonathan.

Family Fun Time

> "The word is Big," says Kate.
> Mom quickly chooses a card from her hand and puts it face down. Jonathan takes a little longer, but soon decides and puts down his choice.

Mom is on the lookout to make sure Kate is patient and sensitive if Jonathan has a hard time choosing.

> Kate mixes up the two cards so she doesn't know who put down each one, then she turns them over.

Mom has watched carefully to make sure Kate mixes the cards well. She wants all to appear fair for Jonathan.

> One card says Mouse, the other says Airplane. Kate gets to judge the best match.
> Kate says, "These are good cards. Big Mouse or Big Airplane. One is funny and one actually makes sense. I like them both!"

Kate really doesn't know who chose which card, so she is careful to compliment both choices. She, too, has learned how to handle some of the interactions during Family Fun Time.

Mom's mind is on another detail: Will Kate choose quickly so that Jonathan does not become impatient?

> Mom uses the running commentary technique to give social information to Jonathan and ease this micro-transition. "Kate is thinking now. She is reading the card and trying to decide which card she likes."
> Kate finally makes her choice. "I choose Mouse."
> "That's mine!" exclaims Jonathan and takes the green card to keep as his point.

Mom realizes that she needs to work on many levels to keep the structure and momentum going, as this seems to help Jonathan feel more comfortable and less stressed. She has learned that her tone of voice is important, and has begun to think of herself as a calm announcer – though mostly in the background – as she keeps track of game details. At the same time, she is a participant in the game. Whether watching or guiding, she is very aware that she holds together the fabric of their interactions.

Relaxing the Structure

At some point I would recommend that Mom relax the structure as Jonathan seems ready. For example, the time between turns could be extended by including more small talk. To make this possible, the concept of small talk needs to be taught, along with social information about when it is appropriate. Monitoring how Jonathan responds to this change in routine is another aspect of the process.

Also keep in mind that while Family Fun Time is initially slanted toward the Autistic child, we have to consider how to balance this out so they are prepared for the world outside of this bubble. Fun Time should evolve to be less slanted as a child moves toward social independence.

Seeing Through Chaos

When is a trivia game more than a trivia game? When it is a golden opportunity to help a child find their footing in our crazy world.

> With only five minutes on the clock, Mom is thinking ahead. There is time for one trivia question per person. Both kids seem to be okay with this. Mom is the one who always asks the questions, and she has a trivia list at hand, fresh from the activities box.
> Mom turns to Kate first, and reads the question: "In which movie does Cruella de Ville appear?" She gives multiple choices so that if someone doesn't know the answer they can guess:
> 1. Lady and the Tramp
> 2. 101 Dalmatians
> 3. Bambi
> 4. Frozen

Mom can see that Jonathan knows the answer and is waiting to let his sister answer first. He is learning to wait for his turn.

Family Fun Time

> Kate knows the answer and says, "#1: Lady and the Tramp."

And that would be the end of this trivia round, except that Mom adds a carefully considered response:

> "Yes, that is what this answer sheet says. Jonathan, do you agree with the answer?"

What is the backstory here? It's this: Jonathan's mom knows from experience that sometimes, albeit rarely, the answers to trivia questions can be wrong. Whether she buys the trivia game at a store or finds the questions online, she knows that misprints, mistakes, and wrong information are all just part of life. We all know this, right? It comes as no surprise. What surprised her was Jonathan's reaction when they encountered a wrong answer during a game. Jonathan didn't usually get upset when he was wrong at trivia, but this time he had a meltdown. He seemed so certain – and got so upset – that Mom did some research and learned that he was actually correct.

What's the big deal? The trivia card had the wrong answer. So what? This will probably never happen again.

Well the big deal is this: Mom had discovered a concept gap. Jonathan did not realize incorrect trivia cards were possible. He couldn't even imagine a mistake like that could exist. And as it turned out, he could not conceive of incorrect information coming from *any* authoritative source, including teachers. Suddenly this explained some of his difficulties at school, where similar meltdowns had occurred, and where things were not always as black and white as a trivia answer. Perceptions of right and wrong vary widely; rules can be illogical and self-contradictory. People are always mistaking facts for opinions, and although it is rare for the teacher's answer book to have the wrong answer, it is not uncommon for answers to be subject to interpretation, and it's very common indeed for the teacher's own logic to be faulty in the eyes of a very literal and logical child. Most of us shrug this stuff off.

> Jonathan responds, "Yes, Mom the answer sheet is correct."

This one simple element in the way they play the game – verifying the answer with Jonathan – may seem like a small thing, yet it is significant. Mom is helping him see through the chaos by validating his experience that the world can seem wrong. By doing so she is helping him on his journey to bridge a concept gap, reinforcing the idea that even authorities make mistakes and that right and wrong are not always so clear cut. Most significantly, she is giving him something solid to trust beyond the chaotic appearance of our social world: his own connection with his mom. No opportunity is too small.

Transitioning Out

> "Okay Jonathan, there is one minute left. Here is your last question..."
>
> Jonathan answers the last question (he gets it right), and now it is time to bring Family Fun Time to a close for the day.

Do you know how endings feel to your child? Endings can feel like a deprivation to some, or even like a punishment. From a traditional viewpoint, one would assume that Jonathan simply will not want to go back to his waiting homework. What child would? But let's not make the mistake of looking at this through neurotypical glasses. Yes, the pending homework might be a factor, but it's not the whole story.

Think of what it's like to lose track of time. You know the feeling: *Oh my, how did it get so late?* Think of the emotional distress of the appointment you'll now miss or the task that will go unfinished, not to mention the sudden shock of realizing that time got away from you. Running out of time is stressful for all of us, and losing track of time can be momentarily quite disorienting. However, when you lose track of time, you know that it is *you* who have lost track. Time marches forward with or without our awareness. When we lose track, we catch up again. You may try to stay ahead of schedule, or feel you are always behind – and time may seem to go by quickly or slowly – but your concept of time remains intact as a phenomenon operating outside of yourself.

Now let's try the *what if* technique from Chapter 12 to imagine what it might be like for Jonathan. Remember, *what if* cannot tell us what a child literally perceives; it's an educated guess to close the compassion gap and give us some reasonable ideas to try.

So...*what if* you had *permanently* lost track of time? More precisely, what if you had no concept of time in the normal "time marches on" sense? All you have is that distressed and disoriented feeling whenever there is a delay or transition. *What if* this is what Jonathan is about to feel when the trivia game ends? How would you make it easier for him?

> *Mom eases into the transition. To make it less abrupt, she offers her son some choices.*
> "It's time for homework now, and I need to cook dinner. Jonathan, do you want to ask me two movie trivia questions while I start dinner, or go straight to homework?"

In the past, Jonathan opted for additional questions. Mom accommodated, but also gave social information such as the following:

👍 *Endings aren't forever.*

👍 *You will play trivia again.*

👍 *There is more time in the future.*

She would also let him write "trivia" on the next Fun Time agenda. Over time Jonathan has realized that everyone in the family operates according to a schedule. He no longer experiences endings as arbitrary punishments, and has become more comfortable with them.

> *Jonathan replies that he would like to do his homework.*
> *Mom says, "Ok, I'll get dinner started and then come see if your teachers are torturing you with homework tonight."*

Jonathan knows that his mother is teasing, and this is another way in which she eases the transition for him. She actually uses something close to sarcasm here, which I generally recommend against. She gets away with it because her remark is not negating. It validates Jonathan's own feelings. This is all a result of doing the necessary preparation. I have seen this level of success with many Autistic children.

I don't want to set unreasonable expectations. Does it always go exactly as I've described? Certainly not. Every child's journey to social independence is difference. My goal is to spark ideas, point out pitfalls, and get your child's journey started. Aim for the possible, and you might find that the possible keeps expanding.

> Mom asks, "What do you want to do next time?"
> Jonathan says, "Show some funny video clips."
> Mom says, "Okay, but let's limit them to four minutes each."
> She jots that down on the agenda for next time and puts it in the activities box. Both children head to their homework areas, and Kate is texting as she goes.

Groundwork for Play Dates

Family Fun Time plants the seeds for play dates. The structure and practice at home prepares your child for more social independence. Plan activities with the possibility of other participants in mind, and think about who might join when your child seems ready and open to the idea. This way the possibility of socializing with other children won't be such a large leap of faith for either you or your child. Start with Family Fun Time, and make it natural to add another child into it.

Family Fun Time is also a way to assess your child's readiness for environments that do not provide the support they get at home. Your child is not going to find all of your accommodations out there in the world. Does this mean you should begin to wean them from your accommodations? Think of it this way: Accommodations bring you more reliable communication. So no, you don't want to go back to *unreliable* communication! You will always want to have more accommodations at home than the outside world will have.

On the other hand, you are preparing your child for broader horizons, starting with play dates. Over time you can wean your child from some of the structure, letting go of accommodations that another parent would not be expected to provide. You also have the option of hosting a play date in your own home, where you can participate and continue to provide all the support that is needed.

21

Social Choreography

When you begin to plan an activity, it is helpful to run through its structure in your head and imagine all the social interactions involved. For some people this can be overwhelming. If it feels that way to you, just imagine how it feels to a child on the autism spectrum. For neurotypical people there is usually a natural rhythm to a game's social interactions. We're not used to breaking down the details. For an Autistic child, it may well be the opposite: all detail and no natural rhythm.

Try this: Observe a group of neurotypical people as they play a game. Look for the rhythm of the interactions. You might not even need to watch them; listening alone reveals the rhythm of a game. One time at a family gathering I listened from another room as family members played a card game that I was not familiar with. The sound of the game progressed through very distinct phases, noticeable even to someone (like me) who did not know the rules. This was like the "social skeleton" of the game. There was chit chat as cards were dealt; quiet periods as players studied their hands and thought about their strategies; rounds of bidding that sounded rather serious; rounds of play punctuated by occasional jokes and laughter. Finally there came a burst of animated discussion as everyone talked about the hand just played. And then the cycle repeated. A most definite social structure had evolved out of the rules of the game, without anyone needing to explain it.

My point? A game's rules might well be within the grasp of an Autistic child, but the social structure is often more elusive. *Why is everyone talking now? Why is everyone quiet now?* Don't assume your child will automatically match the correct social behavior to the flow of a game. (This social awareness is not based on intelligence, by the way. Your child might be a quick study when it comes to strategizing in the "thinking" part of a game, which may lead them to be impatient or bored as everyone else takes more time. A child can lose focus as their own social rhythm falls out of sync with the group.)

The more you pay attention to the social rhythm of an activity, the better able you will be to help your child understand the changing texture of interactions as the activity takes place. That is what I mean by social choreography. Frankly, it is something people seldom think about when planning activities. Do you see its importance?

Even very simple games have a social rhythm. Let's imagine a group playing a simple card game like Go Fish. What if each person began to act out of sync with the rhythm of the game? The dealer deals too slowly. Instead of taking their cards, someone starts a conversation about a favorite movie. Somebody else leaves the table with no explanation. Players question the game: *Why can't I just match the colors? When is it my turn? If this is "Go Fish" then where are the fish?*

Now I'm certainly not saying that Autistic children would do all these things. I'm just trying to highlight some of the social underpinnings of a simple game. The main goal here is to develop a sense of social choreography by understanding the unspoken social rhythms of games and activities. These are rhythms you probably know well, but an Autistic child doesn't. Think of how easy it is for social timing to go awry when things don't happen as they should, when they should. Think of how difficult an activity is for someone who does not know what to do – or, most importantly – why they are doing it.

Thinking in Details

Thinking in details means thinking about *what, why* and *when*. It is not always easy to break down activities to this degree, but it is an effective way to understand an Autistic child's perspective. I don't want to overwhelm you with details. However, I do want you to feel confident that you will eventually be able to manage all the subtleties that lurk in even the simplest activity. Paying attention to details that most people take for granted is one way to discover your child's social blind spots and help them see what they have been missing. That is what social choreography is all about.

Is any activity exempt from social choreography? Not really, not when other people are involved. After all, every interaction is a social interaction.

What about arts and crafts? I have known parents who assumed that their Autistic child would be able to join right in on an art project. After all, art can be rather free-form. It is obviously fun and its value is self-evident, right? Well for some Autistic children this creative endeavor can be more than a little confusing. *Why am I drawing? What am I drawing? What is the point of this? When will it be over?*

The same goes for pretty much any activity. Remember, your activities need to make sense to your child. Think: *why*, *what*, and *when*.

Why Are We Doing This?

Don't assume your child knows that you are just trying to have fun. This may need to be stated rather directly:

> 👍 *Did anyone ever tell you that it is important for families to have fun together? It is doing something all the family members like so we can spend time with each other in a way that's enjoyable for everyone.*

It may turn out that a particular activity is simply not fun for your child. Please do not take it personally. An adolescent on the spectrum might seem disrespectful if a new activity is introduced without explanation. They might even roll their eyes and say, "This is stupid." I realize this is hard to take when you put the effort into creating the rejected activity. Don't give up! This is a chance to prove your value as a social coach by owning the problem.

I would initially respond in a very calm manner, being careful not to use a sarcastic tone (even if your child does):

> 👍 *I tried to pick an activity that would be fun for the family. If I picked the wrong activity, then clearly I did a bad job! The purpose is to have fun, not to annoy you. It is important for families to have fun together. I will try to pick better activities. Thank you for being nice to me while I do this.*

Your child might not even realize that planning a fun family activity is possible. Maybe fun activities are so rare that your child has given up on the idea. Picking an activity that is actually enjoyable for your child flips things around so you don't have to explain why you are doing it. It is worth doing some detective work to find out what is fun for them, and why. You can use close-ended questions:

👍 *Would you like to play Bingo or a trivia game about Star Wars? Which is better?*

Be sure they are aware that "I don't know" is an okay answer.

It Depends

When asking a child about preferences, I also like to offer "It depends" as a choice. Your child might not *always* pick Bingo over trivia. It might depend on their mood, what they played yesterday, who will play, what rules will be used, how much time there will be. *It depends* is a really valuable choice that may lead to insights into why your child likes what they like.

If your child is resistant to participating in *any* activities, then ask them to just watch at first. After they watch you can ask if the activity seemed good or dumb. Again, try not to take their feedback personally. I know this can be hard!

What Will You Do If...?

The "what" part of activity planning does not just refer to what activity you'll do in general – it refers to what you will do at each step along the way. What will we do if this happens? What will we do if that happens? Whether or not your child has questions along these lines, you need to be asking *yourself* these questions so you can choreograph smooth social interactions if any of the contingencies occur.

The more you take the time to imagine each part of an activity, the better prepared you will be to avoid bad surprises and general confusion. It's easy to underestimate the amount of "pre-imagining" that is required. For example, in our case study in the previous chapter, the family played a game of trivia. The mom did not just jot down trivia questions on a list without further planning. Well, maybe she tried this at first, then experience taught her better. Trial-and-error is indeed one way to learn the amount of pre-planning you will need. Of course we'd like to minimize the error side of the equation in order to reduce stress all around. Still, let's not be paranoid about mistakes. Accommodations should give you confidence to deal with any missteps. This is a learning process that needs to run its course.

If you can answer questions like the following, you will be in pretty good shape. The idea is to deconstruct any activity into these kinds of "what will you do if..." questions. These questions are based on the trivia game example, but this type of contingency thinking can be applied to any activity. The questions alone reveal the social choreography of the game.

➤ **What will you do if** your child is not interested in the activity? This mom specifically played movie trivia, her son's favorite topic. At this stage she gears the activities toward his interests. What is interesting to *your* child?

➤ **What will you do if** your child cannot do part of the activity? In our example, Mom read the trivia questions instead of having her children take turns reading. Some children might prefer to read the questions themselves. In this case, think about what questions they'll get to read. Will some be too hard? Do you need to choose in advance? What type of questions will you pick?

➤ **What will you do if** your child has difficulty answering the questions? Some children have a very difficult time when they answer wrong. If this is the case, then trivia might not be the best choice. Mom gave multiple choice answers so her son could guess if he didn't know an answer. What will work in your case? Maybe hints should be part of the game. What hints will you give?

➤ **What will you do if** your child cannot handle losing? Mom did not keep score. For her son, this was the best plan. What kind of scorekeeping will you do?

➢ **What will you do if** your child has a hard time with transitions? The mom in our example had waiting activities for transitioning in and out of the activity. What waiting activities will you have available?

Let me pause to reassure you that this level of planning does not happen overnight. You may already know answers to some of these questions; others will become clear as your lines of communication improve. You will no doubt identify more "what will you do if..." questions as you try out different activities.

Here are more examples of social choreography from the trivia game in the previous chapter:

➢ Mom knew what to do if the trivia game printed the wrong answer (or if her child *thought* the answer was wrong).

➢ Mom knew what to do if the phone rang.

➢ Mom knew what to do if her son answered out of turn.

➢ Mom knew what to do if time was running short.

Is this overkill? Well, if it's making your head spin, take a break from the dance and don't worry about it. I don't want this level of detail to stop you from trying. Mainly, I want you to be aware that all these details exist, whether or not you are able to plan for them in advance. When and if an unexpected contingency pops up, at least now you can think: *Ah, so this is what that book meant by 'social choreography!'*

Choreograph as much as you can to the degree that it's comfortable for you. For me, the planning lets me relax. Although I'm good at improvising in the moment, some solid advance planning assures that I am always a beat or two ahead. I always have something at my fingertips when things don't go as I'd hoped. It's my job, after all, and I get plenty of practice dealing with the unexpected. My advice to parents: Plan to the point where you feel confident about what to do in some likely situations. Do not plan to the point where you worry about everything that *might* go wrong. In other words, don't let the planning stifle the joy of interacting with your child. If anything goes awry, you're certain to learn some new choreography for next time.

When Do I Do Something?

Most any activity involves timing. When will it start? When does it end? When is it my turn? Don't assume that your child automatically knows this information, even if it seems obvious to you. *Especially* if it seems obvious to you.

Questions of *when* arise along with the *what* aspect of a game. In a trivia game, someone asks questions, and others answer. Your child may wonder: *So when do I get to ask a question? When do I get to answer? When is there a winner? How do we know when to stop?*

A child might be eager to participate: *When do I get to do something?* You don't necessarily need to explain everything in advance. You can lead the game one step at a time:

👍 *I will ask the first question, and you answer first.*

A more fearful child might be afraid of making a misstep. They might wonder: *When do I have to do something?* Reassure them, even if they leave the question unspoken:

👍 *I will tell you what to do when it is time.*

Knowing when to stop is another sensitive area for children on the spectrum. I always like to announce the ending before we get there:

👍 *One more question, then we're done.*

Card games and board games usually have a well-defined structure, and of course these all have questions of *when*: *When do I deal the cards? When do I roll the dice? When do I lose a turn?*

Again, explain as you go:

👍 *I will tell you when it is your turn. I will tell you when to show your cards.*

There are other, more subtle rhythms to games. For example, some games have "think time" when the players need to sort cards or quietly consider their next play. The quiet time is part of the social interaction. More questions of *when*: *When can I talk? When should I be quiet? When should I sit still? When can I get up for a snack?*

Be sensitive to the fact that your child will not necessarily ask such questions, or even be aware of these considerations. The unspoken social choreography exists for everyone else, but not for those who can't perceive the rhythm.

Try to anticipate confusion before it happens:

👍 *It is time to be quiet and look at your cards. Put the same colors together.*

Even so-called unstructured activities raise questions of *when*. As I mentioned earlier, arts and crafts need more structure than you might think. If you're going to do a particular project, it helps to have a finished sample and a good idea of how long it will take your child to complete it. Again, those questions of timing: *When do I use the paint? When do I glue on the ribbon? What if I run out of time?*

So many questions! You might be wondering: is a simple activity really this confusing to my child? For many children the answer is *yes*.

Autistic children will often have questions like these, even if they don't know how to ask. The questions may be little more than a sense of unease from not knowing what will happen next. Some children will wonder about the structure of an activity, while others will not know that activities even have a structure. It may feel like a child is challenging the routine, when in reality they just don't understand that there *is* a routine. If you don't know when you've done something wrong and find you're being corrected all the time, that's kind of a big problem. It's hard to have fun under such conditions.

What questions will your child ask? What should be explained even if your child doesn't ask? I'm trying to make you aware of all these *potential* questions so you can stay a step ahead.

I'm sorry if absorbing all these details seems like studying for a test, but the analogy fits. To be well prepared, you need to know more than the test will cover. At least in this test, close is often good enough. And

Social Choreography

you'll get to take the test again and again.

You don't need to think of everything in advance (although the more the better). And you certainly don't want to subject your child to a 30 minute lecture before playing a card game – that kind of information overload can be very disorienting, especially if your child doesn't understand why you are explaining so much. On the other hand, if your child asks lots of questions, then by all means give them specific information:

👍 *I will go first, then your sister will go, then it will be your turn.*

Or they might be looking for general reassurance. Then you can say:

👍 *I will help you know what to do. It's okay to watch before you play.*

Have accommodations ready when you need them. This does not just mean picture schedules, problem scales, silent timers, and other tangible items – although I strongly recommend these. It also means knowing how to adjust your language, how to put facts before feelings, how to own misunderstandings, and generally how to tune the techniques in this book to your child's specific needs. The most important accommodation is your own intent to help your child feel safe and understood.

22

Components of Social Independence

I tell parents of Autistic children not to give their child more social freedom than they can responsibly handle. You don't want to set your child up for failure. Social failures are a sure way to diminish self-esteem and self-confidence. Our goal is to maximize social freedom and independence, but we also want your child to be physically and emotionally safe.

I know parents who have pushed their children to join scouts or community events with the hope that social skills would emerge. Sadly, this can lead to meltdowns and tears. If you take a step back, I bet you can make a good prediction about how your child will fare. Past behavior is the best predictor of future success. Don't push your child to join the kids playing outside if you don't think it will work. First assess. Is your child ready to navigate the social interactions?

Now don't get me wrong, I'm not saying never try, but be aware of the risks. Remember the boy who was asked to choose just one toy? (See *The True or False Game* in Chapter 6.) You could say he was given more social freedom than he could handle with just a simple decision to make at home. A basic concept gap tripped him up, and he did not have the tools to clarify the situation on his own. However, his parents were there with the tools to help him. That is a beginning.

My point is that you can take more risks in situations that you control. Dare greatly! But stay within the bounds of what your child can safely handle. How do you know those bounds? Well, if you have breezed past the Family Fun Time idea, please go back and consider one of its tremendous benefits: it's a custom laboratory in which you can evaluate the amount of social freedom that your child is ready for.

> **No Need for Apologies**
>
> To strike the right balance as you help your child expand their horizons outside the home, you need to find an honest answer to one more question about letting them participate in social situations: is your caution due to their emotional needs, or yours?
>
> Some parents feel self-conscious about their children. I have been in many social situations with Autistic children whose parents have apologized to me on their behalf for some unusual behavior or another. But this I feel strongly: a child's right to be out in the world should not be limited because they might appear unusual to others. There is no need to apologize – especially to me! I'm not at all uncomfortable. I do understand that society is not always so accepting, which is why you may initially need to create environments in which you are comfortable and your child feels safe; for example, by planning a play date...the topic of the next chapter.
>
> If you are uncomfortable seeing your child's attempts to socialize, then make that your motivation to help. Be cautious about risks when it comes to your child's well-being, but don't hold them back because of your own discomfort.

I've used the phrase "social independence" quite a bit. This chapter explains its important components, and shows how the accommodations you've learned can be used to build these important areas:

➢ Valid reporting

➢ Accepting feedback

➢ Self-observation

➢ Effective self-advocacy

➢ Independent social learning

Let's take a closer look.

Valid Reporting

What does valid reporting look like? A young neurotypical boy might run to a parent crying if his older brother teases him. Parents then ask questions, get reliable answers (if the boy isn't being deceitful), and help solve the problem. Do you see how the child's point of view is being accurately represented? Even if he is being deceitful, a point of view has been deliberately conveyed. He is doing it on purpose. The child's intent is telegraphed accurately.

However, things can be quite different with a child on the autism spectrum. Their point of view is not represented in a way that others understand in any kind of dependable fashion, yet often no one is aware of this. A child is silent, and we assume nothing is wrong. A child speaks calmly, and we assume they are not upset. A child has a meltdown, and we say that it's a behavior to be discouraged. They have not represented their point of view in a way we understand, and neither party seems to be aware that the miscommunication has occurred.

What is involved here? There are questions of what should be reported, and to whom. There is the challenge of getting the facts on the table in as neutral a way as possible before we even begin to think about solving a problem or teaching a lesson. Without valid reporting, there is a disconnection between what help we think is needed, and the help that is actually needed. Often there is a discrepancy between a child's ability to observe outer facts and their less developed capacity to observe their own actions and reactions.

And then there is the matter of concept gaps. A child on the spectrum will not perceive the same objective world as you. How big are the differences? Does the child understand the need to describe their own experience? Do they see the value in conversations about their everyday life? Perhaps the child believes their point of view is automatically seen and understood by everyone, because after all, how could there possibly be more than one point of view? Imagine how inexplicable our behavior is to a child with a fundamental misunderstanding about the very existence of misunderstandings.

Here's an example:

Many children on the spectrum have sensory integration issues. Heightened senses can cause a child to become confused, distressed, and even angry. Sound, light, motion, smells, and tactile sensations can all trigger sensory overload in some children. Now here's the deeper problem: not all children can accurately report these issues. It would be ideal if a child could say, "Music class is too hard for me because the piano is so loud when the teacher plays that it hurts my brain, and I feel like I need to run out of the room." However, we don't usually see this level of reporting. You'll generally get the behavior without the explanation.

So why doesn't the child explain their experience? Every child is different. I have found a variety of reasons that apply to a situation like this. At the one end of the continuum you are dealing with a basic lack of social skills. The child doesn't know they can report their difficultly, or is unaware of how to do it. Often there is a bigger obstacle: a lack of trust that anyone can help. No call for help has ever worked before, so why should this time be different? Further along the continuum, the child may believe that they *have* asked for help (after all, they ran from the room), but asking for help *that* way has only met with punishment, another miscommunication due to lack of valid reporting.

At the far end of the continuum, you will find a much more surprising viewpoint. I can tell you that some children literally do not know that they are the only ones experiencing the distress. For them the intolerable situation is doubly disorienting because nobody else is acting appropriately. *Why is the teacher torturing our eardrums? Why isn't everybody blocking their ears and running from the room? This is a 911 emergency! Where are the police?*

Who would *you* trust in this upside-down world? Let's see what we can do about this kind of situation.

Nurture Valid Reporting

I've tried to show you many benefits of the accommodations in this book. Here's one more: they help nurture valid reporting. Consider the following specific applications:

- ➢ **Keep the conversation going.** Demonstrate the value of talking about daily events. All of the Facts Before Feelings accommodations in Chapter 6 are aimed at creating an open and enjoyable communication channel. In your conversations, unreported issues will come to light.

Components of Social Independence

> **The 1-5 scales** (Chapter 8) can help uncover your child's views on many topics. Together with a neutral fact-based communication style, you can get to the bottom of situations that distress your child. Get the problem on the table.

> **The "Did anyone ever tell you"** technique (chapter 13) can be useful to explain about sensory issues, and pretty much any problem your child reports. Does your child know why they are the only one bothered by the piano playing? Own the oversight for never explaining before.

> **A problem jar** (Chapter 16) is an extremely useful tool to foster valid reporting. The "loud piano" problem goes in the jar, and Mom and Dad help come up with a solution. Earplugs, noise-canceling headphones, a planned escape route (*I have talked to the teacher and she will let you wait outside the classroom*) – these can all be part of a "bad surprise" plan for days when the teacher feels musically inclined.

Accommodations illuminate your child's world. At first you are the one to initiate their use, but accommodations also give your child a way to explain their point of view. From the very moment you start using them, you are showing your child something basic and extremely important: you are showing that they have a point of view, it is valid, and it is possible to express it. This is the "understanding" part of *safe and understood*. You not only help them feel understood – you show them it is *possible* to feel understood.

Quantify the Environment

Here is a more subtle way in which you can help a child report their experiences. The goal is for your child to become aware of the environment and the way it affects them. This requires some sensitivity on your part to recognize the sensitivities of your child. We'll continue with the example of sound sensitivity, but the appraoch can apply to many of your child's experiences.

Consider how a music therapist can quantify sounds in the environment by demonstrating the loudness of her guitar before she plays:

The Connection Formula

👍 *My guitar will not get any louder than this.*

She could sing at the maximum volume she plans to use:

👍 *My singing will not get louder than this.*

For parents who don't sing or play music, the approach still applies:

👍 *My voice will get this loud when I laugh or when I talk over other people to give a safety warning. Here is how it sounds when I clap my hands.*

How does this help with valid reporting? It demonstrates the parameters that are quantifiable in the environment. What types of sound are harder to tolerate? Is it volume, pitch, conflicting sounds (such as too many people talking at once), or sudden sounds? Observe a child's responses to sensory input and help them to become aware of how they are affected. The goal is for the child to figure out what is overwhelming and what is tolerable. Don't assume they automatically know. Sorting sounds in the environment and labeling them makes their experience of sound seem a little less random.

Your child may eventually be able to do this themselves, but as you get started, you do all the quantifying. This can lead to some practical problem solving as they learn to recognize the specific source of their distress. Try to quantify the environment by labeling and categorizing.

For sensitivity to smells:

👍 *I will never bring food into the room without telling you first.*

👍 *I will not wear perfume.*

👍 *I will not use that cheese you do not like.*

For light sensitivity:

👍 *I will only turn one light on.*

Components of Social Independence

- 👍 *Do you want me to turn the overhead lights on? Or do you want me to leave them off?*
- 👍 *I have covered the switch with tape so nobody will turn on the bright light while you are in the room.*

For tactile sensitivity:

- 👍 *I will not touch you without permission.*
- 👍 *You can decide which chair is the most comfortable.*
- 👍 *Different clothing has different feelings. Some have a good feeling and some have a bad feeling. I don't know how your body feels in these new clothes. You can rate the clothes on a 1-5 scale.*

Tactile sensitivity is particularly tricky when family members want to hug your child. Even people who sit too close can make a child uncomfortable.

* * *

It can be easy to think that someone with sensory issues is just over-reacting if you have not experienced such sensitivities yourself. The problem really can be quite stressful. Many unexplained behaviors might be due to just such an issue. By giving voice to these matters yourself, you aim to give your child a voice so they can report on the problem independently.

Can this approach be applied to other issues? Let's see. Remember Elliot, the boy in Chapter 12 who would run up to the whiteboard to correct the teacher's mistake? Sensitivity to mistakes can be just as difficult as sensory issues for some children, and can be much harder for a neurotypical person to understand. It may stem from the need to make order and predictability in the environment. The boy's attention is much more on some minor mistake than the social choreography of the classroom. The rhythm of the classroom eludes him, while the mistake is glaring and obvious.

How does one "quantify the environment" for a sensitivity like this?

I've already given you some techniques that apply here. First, own any misunderstandings. This is the essence of the "Did anyone ever tell you" technique. The technique is intended to protect your child emotionally when it comes to their own mistakes and social missteps. Normalize the idea that mistakes exist in the world. I will often use the phrase, "Oh, that was my mistake." Or: "I made a mistake with my words." This won't magically reduce a child's aversion to mistakes; more work might be needed. Our goal here is to create a framework in which mistakes are seen as normal so that your child will have a context for understanding and reporting their experiences regarding this sensitivity.

Another approach worth remembering is the idea of allowing a child to point out your mistakes. I've mentioned that I do this in my socialization groups. It's not a technique for everyone or every situation, but it can help move things forward.

We hope to reach a greater level of self-observation regarding the sensitivity. What if the child could say:

> "I know this might be a little random, but you misspelled the author's name and he is one of my favorite authors. I read his book three times and I'm a bit obsessed. Sorry for the interruption, but if someone searched for his name the way you spelled it, they would not get the right hits."

And I would say, "That makes perfect sense, thanks for telling me."

This example may be unrealistic, and even if a child on the spectrum put things so clearly, it might still be off-putting. You won't be able to change how others see this type of self-expression, but at home you can strive to quantify and normalize any area that needs improved lines of communication. I would consider anything close to this level of reporting a great step forward for many children whose motivation has been misunderstood for so long.

If It's New, First Review

We have discussed what it is to be a valid reporter. Now let's address the question of knowing what needs to be reported, and when. I try to teach children this rule of thumb: *If it's new, first review.* I explain that whenever something new or unusual comes up, review it with your parents.

Components of Social Independence

Let's say your teen agreed to provide snacks at an after school club and never told you. He is getting ready for school on the day of the event when he lets you know. Or maybe he never lets you know! Everyone is depending on him, but he shows up empty-handed. Letting you know about a commitment is a slightly different angle on valid reporting. If your child learns that *when it's new, first review*, you might have a chance to find out about a potential commitment before it is made. Your teen can learn to respond to requests by saying, "I don't know if I can do that. I'll let you know." Then he will have a chance to review the plan with you.

Valid reporting is very important when your child is bullied or put at risk in some way. I read an article about a teen on the spectrum who was arrested because an undercover agent in the high school "caught" him dealing drugs in an elaborate sting operation. According to the article, the teen was befriended by the undercover agent who then encouraged him to acquire some drugs. The article explained that the teen did not have any involvement with drugs prior to this, but was very enthusiastic about his new "friend." I do not know all the details of the case, but I can imagine how far in over his head this teen was. I can also imagine that the agent did not have the teen's best interest at heart; neither would any so-called "real" friend who wanted to involve someone in drugs. How is a teen on the autism spectrum equipped to judge the authenticity of a friendship? This teen was truly in a situation where he was given more social freedom than he could responsibly handle. Scenarios like this certainly raise the stakes for knowing when to report information.

Would a policy of *when it's new, first review* have kept this teen out of trouble? Possibly, if he was able to follow through. You can see why it's so important to keep the lines of communication open.

Knowing when to report information can be very confusing for someone on the spectrum. Should your child report every minor infraction they see, like a classmate texting in class or chewing gum when it is against the rules? If a child tells on people too much it does not work in their favor. How are they to know what to report, when to report it, and what to let go? *When it's new, first review* is a useful rule of thumb for the minimum amount to report. I would rather your child report too much information – to *you* – than not enough. Yes, I know this might keep you very busy, but at least the topic of your child's daily life will stay up front and center.

Good communication is not just for a crisis; you want a communication channel open all the time. This is clearly sound advice for neurotypical children as well. For Autistic children, it requires accommodations to make conversations about everyday life accessible.

Accepting Feedback

Parenting requires teaching your child about life. You guide them from the moment they are born. You encourage them to share their toys when they are young. You make sure they do their homework. When they are teenagers you teach them how to drive a car and make good decisions. You give them feedback in response to their actions to help improve the quality of their lives.

People have different responses to feedback, depending on their temperament and how the feedback is given. My observation is that most people do not enjoy getting direct feedback because it feels like criticism. Too much critical feedback has a negative impact on self-esteem. Instead of motivating someone to accept your insights and guidance, just the opposite happens. A harsh critique can be demoralizing. Also, the person giving the feedback becomes the bad guy.

How does this apply to an Autistic child striving for social independence? Just think of all the focus put on teaching social skills to children on the spectrum: when to speak, when to be silent; saying "please" and "thank you"; proper table manners – countless rules and their tangle of exceptions. There is even feedback about making eye contact! If all of this information is perceived as criticism, then why would anyone be open to it? On the other hand, when a child truly needs social information, how do we ensure that it is well-received?

Our goal is for them to accept information about their social interactions without feeling defeated or devalued. And so we give feedback in a supportive manner.

However, you are not your child's only source of feedback. They receive feedback from peers, from teachers, from other family members, and from the community. These people will not all be using The Connection Formula. Where does this leave us? If your child talks about one topic for too long, a friend might tell them that they're boring. How will your child handle feedback like that? Will they listen? Will they ignore it? Will they see its value?

If a child is good at receiving feedback, they might say something like this: "Sorry, thanks for letting me know," and then change the subject. Ideally, they would not feel insulted. They would view this as important information rather than criticism. (I am imagining in this scenario that the friend is really a friend and not just a rude acquaintance or someone with questionable motives – although such a graceful response might work regardless.) Meanwhile, back in the real world, we all know that accepting feedback gracefully is easier said than done. Being so gracious even just once in a while is a great accomplishment. More often, especially for a child on the autism spectrum, the feedback is confusing, hurtful, or just plain irrelevant, and so it has no positive effect.

The more you can provide supportive feedback at home, the more you prepare your child for the wider world. First, your child may be able to sidestep some of the harsher criticisms if you are able to fill a concept gap at home:

👍 *Oh, didn't anyone ever tell you that not everybody has the same interest about a topic? You can say three things about a topic, and then stop to hear what the other person says about the thoughts in their head.*

Second, your child may be able to build more resilience to feedback when they can see the value of it. Think of it this way: there is a feedback-to-value ratio. If the feedback makes no sense (as perceived by your child), then it has no relevance and hence no value. If the feedback is painful to hear, then its sting outweighs its value. The cumulative effect of hurtful feedback is obviously negative, and can leave an Autistic child feeling afraid of life. But if the feedback is given in a way that is meaningful and does not wound your child, then they will be more likely to apply it. This increases self-confidence along with the perceived value of the feedback.

We want the cumulative effect of feedback to be positive. There is no guarantee that any particular child will build resilience to outside criticism, but you certainly improve the chances when your work at home has put your child's self-confidence on the rise. Consistently supportive feedback received from trusted people like parents and counselors will allow your child to navigate new social situations, and this leads to less fear and more trust in life.

The ability to accept feedback while maintaining emotional balance is a very important skill for an Autistic child – and indeed, for anyone – to develop. It opens the door to mutual understanding. For a child on the autism spectrum, it is the gateway to independent social learning.

Self-Observation

Self-observation is closely connected to accepting feedback. Anyone who has tried to initiate some type of personal change recognizes how challenging it can be. Imagine you are on a weight loss program; this requires you to watch your eating habits. You may discover new things about yourself, for example, that you eat more when under stress. This is self-observation. Now how would it feel if someone else started commenting on your eating habits? That might sting a little, or that might sting a lot! It might even cause stress that leads to more eating – a self-defeating cycle.

Now let's compound the experience by imagining you don't realize that people can self-observe. In other words, you literally don't know what it means to "watch what you are doing." Yet now you receive feedback from others who are able to watch what you do. I know this seems like some kind of brainteaser, but it just might be what life is like for some people on the spectrum. It's a strange world in which you're never sure what others can observe in you that you can't observe in yourself.

For this reason, a child's attention should be brought to self-observation with as little sting as possible. It is best to start your child out by observing other people. The "Who in this family" game is ideal for this. I introduced the game in Chapter 20 as a way to keep things moving during Family Fun Time. To play the game, come up with some easy questions:

👍 *Who in this family...is wearing red sneakers?*

Components of Social Independence

👍 *Who in this family...has four legs and a tail?*

Some questions might require a bit more observation:

👍 *Who in this family...talks on the phone the most?*

The game is a great waiting activity, and it has a deeper benefit: in some cases, the child will answer, "Me!" Do you see? It's a bridge to self-observation.

The Running Commentary technique (Chapter 6) is another great tool to foster self-observation. Go back into the Accommodations part of the book and have a look. You'll see that this technique involves observational comments...neutral statements that compare and contrast, label your feelings (as a way to help your child recognize their own feelings), and explain the behavior of others. Some attention is put on the child; much is put on the world around them. Always this is done in a neutral fashion. So you see, we've been building toward self-observation right from the beginning.

The very notion of self-observation can be a concept gap, so the techniques and accommodations such as, "Didn't anyone ever tell you?", "What's the bigger problem game?", and "The problem pyramid" take this into consideration by gradually bringing attention to it – without the sting.

These strategies give a child a way to observe their own thoughts and feelings, and then provide an avenue to express them. And if done correctly, such accommodations encourage the process of self-observation because the benefits of the process are demonstrated in a way your child understands. For social independence you really want your child on board the self-observation train.

Effective Self-Advocacy

Effective self-advocacy requires one to learn how the world works and understand how it will respond.

Frank, a young man diagnosed Asperger's, did not like the equipment ordering procedure at a computer club where he volunteered. He sent an email about the matter to everyone on the mailing list, expressing in great detail his views on the illogical process. What was the result? Frank was warned that any further "email flames" would get him ejected from the club.

Frank was shocked and upset. He had not intended to "flame" anyone. Not only did his self-advocacy fail to fix the original problem, it created a whole new problem that he did not understand. He had certainly made his views known. Isn't that valid reporting? What went wrong?

Effective self-advocacy involves expressing yourself in a way that will be well-received by others in order to get a problem solved. It can be difficult for all of us. For Frank, it was a complete mystery. He was unaware of how his views would be received by others. But why?

Well, Frank lacked self-observation skills. He focused on the logical aspects of the problem, not his own emotional distress. He could have said, "I personally find this procedure illogical and confusing. I wonder if there's something we can do about it, and I have some suggestions..." Instead, he focused outwardly with a critique of the procedure, and his logic expanded to imply criticism of the club leadership behind it. This all came across as angry and imbalanced. He had put his strong emotions into his email for everyone else to see without being fully aware of those emotions himself.

Now I don't want to say Frank was completely unaware of his emotions. He certainly knew about his discomfort with the club's procedure. It's just that for him it was more natural to focus on logic. The logic felt more relevant than the emotions. And here lies another gap in Frank's self-advocacy skills: he assumed that everyone else would focus solely on the logic, too. If this is how your mind works, why wouldn't you assume that everyone else thinks this way?

Feedback would tell you otherwise.

To nurture good self-advocacy skills, it's important to start early with supportive feedback.

👍 *Oh, didn't anyone ever tell you that not everybody focuses on logic? Many people focus on feelings more than logic.*

If feedback feels positive, then a child is more likely to seek it. The guideline of *when it's new, first review* depends on a child's comfort level with feedback. And this guideline carries naturally into adulthood. What if Frank had thought, *Oh, new situation* – and asked a friend for feedback before sending his email? He might have received some helpful suggestions to keep himself in better standing with the other club members.

So you see, self-observation and the ability to accept feedback are important building blocks for effective self-advocacy.

There is one more piece: understanding cause and effect. The goal of self-advocacy is to achieve a specific result, so obviously cause and effect come into play. Some areas of cause and effect are very elusive to people on the spectrum, often because their underlying concepts and priorities don't match up with the neurotypical viewpoint. In Frank's case, he discounted the effect of emotions and missed the concept that others will prioritize differently. We need to align a child's understanding of cause and effect with the social norms they will encounter throughout life.

Part of self-advocacy is knowing when to ask for help. First, one has to recognize that help may be needed, which comes down to asking the right questions. In Frank's case, it might look like this:

Oh, I'm feeling emotional about this situation; others might focus on my emotions and miss my logic. What effect will that have?

If he can't work out the answer on his own, he will at least know to privately ask for help in the right area and avoid making a very public social misstep.

We want to help Autistic children get their point across. We want them to be heard. We take the initiative by using accommodations to show how communication works. Our accommodations become the child's skills. For adults, these skills are going to present themselves as the ability to problem solve appropriately in a work environment and in relationships. That is effective self-advocacy.

Independent Social Learning

Self-advocacy goes hand-in-hand with independent social learning. Our goal is for these to move forward together. Social learning means learning how to solve problems, manage novel situations, and create friendships – just to name a few areas beyond the basic ability to connect with others and enjoy life.

For someone with a social learning disability, social learning does not take place automatically. If a child on the spectrum is thrown into a social situation without preparation, they can be traumatized by the experience. On the other hand, with the right preparation and support, each successful experience will build on the last until social learning begins to come more naturally. Social independence happens step-by-step, not all at once.

Here are a few basic characteristics to look for:

- ☐ Ability to negotiate plans with others.
- ☐ Ability to deal with the unexpected
- ☐ Ability to figure out what to do in new social situations without relying on a memorized response
- ☐ Ability to interact with others without being afraid or overwhelmed

Social independence ultimately requires the ability to self-learn and move forward on one's own. Not every interaction in life is fun, but social independence gives you more access to fun...and to freedom. The socially independent individual is not paralyzed by fear.

Here's a brief success story:

A co-ed group of five Autistic teenagers went to the mall for a social outing. The group had previously been on many highly structured outings with parents close by. Prior to that, they had gone out as part of their socialization groups. In short, there had been a lot of preparation – years of preparation in some cases. Now on this latest excursion, parents would wait in the food court while the teens went to shop and explore the mall independently.

Shopping in a mall can be a rather unstructured activity. What stores should the group go into? How should they manage their time and money? How will these decisions be made? Parents and children negotiated the duration of the outing. Each teen knew how much money they could spend. Before leaving the food court, the teenagers agreed on which stores they would visit, in what order, and how long they would stay in each one.

Then the group struck out on their own.

As it turned out, one of the stores was very loud, causing a sensory issue for one of the teens. Together they came up with a solution. The teen with the sensory issues stayed outside and another one stayed with him, while the remaining three went in. All five were very proud of this decision and it worked out very well.

For some teens on the spectrum, this unexpected situation could have been very confusing and stressful. The group did not have a prepared plan for it, nor did they have any past experience with this specific scenario. What they did have were some problem solving skills and the ability to express their feelings, so they managed to independently resolve a tricky little social situation.

Some people might think that going to the mall is a socially easy activity. Well that is not necessarily so. In this case I thought the teens had developed the ability to handle the situation and were ready to enjoy a new level of social freedom. Parents agreed, and the teens proved us right.

* * *

Social independence needs to be accomplished in small, manageable pieces. If you are going out to a restaurant and want your ten-year-old son to order directly from the server, where do you begin? You need to know the answer to questions like these:

- ☐ Is he aware of the goal?
- ☐ Is he on board with it?
- ☐ Does it make sense to him?
- ☐ Do you have a reliable way of communicating social expectations?
- ☐ Are you able to consistently communicate the reasons behind the expectations?
- ☐ Does he have a way to communicate his feelings?

If your answer is yes to all of these questions, then it is time to address the goal.

Finding the Right Pace

Knowing when and where to push your child socially is not something that comes naturally. Usually people push too hard, and in the wrong areas. Instead of pushing, think of how you can lead, guide, and encourage.

I need to make it clear that this may be a slower process than you are hoping for. It can take more time than you'd like, but I guarantee it is time well spent. If your child is motivated to move forward socially then we want to keep up that motivation. To do so, you have to move at a pace that allows social successes to outweigh social missteps.

In order to keep our ten-year-old motivated to place his own order, I would be very low-key with the goal. Don't make it a big deal (unless he wants you to do so). It's important to know your child's resilience. If you push too hard, then they might retreat and "go underground." By that I mean that they might lose interest in even trying to socialize.

Use common sense and break things down logically. For example, go to a restaurant your child is familiar with. Try to think of the details. Do they have a preferred order? Make sure the menu hasn't changed. Be a social coach, but again, don't make a big deal out of it. Ask your child what they want to have, but ask others at the table too, so your child doesn't feel singled out.

When the server comes you can give your own order and then ask your child, "Do you want to say your order or do you want me to?" A lack of response probably means that they want you to take over. If they do order then just be very relaxed about it as sometimes too much attention creates or increases anxiety. You can give a thumbs-up or say "good job ordering." If your child wants the attention, then feel free to pour on the positives!

Seeing the Pain

Helping a child on the autism spectrum to be socially independent is transformative work, and it is not just the child who is transformed. This sort of work requires empathy and compassion beyond the norm. I'll end this chapter with a rather subtle story to illustrate.

Components of Social Independence

One day I had to come up with a new seating arrangement for a particular group activity in order to smooth a planned transition. Whenever there are changes, I try to let the children know ahead of time. I don't want them to walk into a new arrangement without prior knowledge, because it could be confusing and disorienting to some of them. I had name tags for the chairs to minimize confusion, but that was not going to be enough. A child on the autism spectrum often needs advance preparation. So when the first of the children arrived in our waiting room, I immediately explained about the changes she would encounter.

How did she react? She asked, "Will you tell me where to sit?"

And I responded, "Yes."

Now you might be thinking *okay...that is a rather simple story*. And so it would seem, yet there is much more to it than meets the eye. To begin with, it's a matter of seeing the pain.

I know how hard change can be for Autistic people. I can see the pain this creates. At times I feel it. It is not just an intellectual concept to me. I am not only thinking about neurological differences related to autism – I am imagining the person with the differences. I am brought to tears even as I write this.

When this young client asked, "Will you tell me where to sit?" I had a glimpse into her world. I knew she asked the question because she was uneasy about the situation. Although I would never make a big deal out of sitting in the "wrong" seat, the possibility of such a mistake still loomed in her mind. The reliable room arrangement was no longer so reliable. We could be looking at a high stress level (a three or above) on a 1-5 scale. Yet her tone of voice was matter-of-fact. She did not sound nervous. Neurotypical perception said, *all is well, no pain in sight*. Yet even though her response would be considered rote by some, I *heard* her. I had seen her pain many times before, and was very sensitized to her viewpoint.

I know that the vast majority of neurotypical people do not relate to the emotional pain that someone with autism experiences. Yes, they see the symptoms. Yes, they might be able to write a social/emotional goal, something along the lines of increasing flexibility with routines. Truly seeing the pain, however, is something of a different sort entirely, a quality that's hard to slice, dice, and quantify. It's of the heart.

The Connection Formula

If you have followed the ideas I've presented, then you know why seeing the pain is so difficult. It's because our perception of what is happening is not commensurate with the child's reality. An Autistic child does not present their reality in terms that resonate with our neurotypical sensibilities; therefore, our interpretation of their needs is inaccurate. In a nutshell, the neurotypical adults think they see all there is to see, but they are oh so wrong.

"Will you tell me where to sit?"

I saw her pain in this question, but there was something else, a very hopeful sign. She was able to ask the question. It showed confidence and the ability to get her needs met. That is self-advocacy, and it is significant. She had asked for help.

As adults, we should want to more accurately perceive the child's reality. The more a child can help us understand their world, the easier it is for both parties. When perception and reality align, then we have closed the compassion gap. You'll know this has happened when you see a child's pain.

There is one more layer to this story. When I simply answered *yes*, I could feel she believed me. She trusted me. She knows I am true to my word. I respect and honor how she perceives things, and she knows that about me. I had proven that to her time and time again.

You might ask: If rearranging the room was so stressful, why did I do it? Wasn't there another way to plan things? Well the change was needed to accommodate an activity that the children were looking forward to. (I wouldn't make an arbitrary change for the sake of change alone.) And there was not much risk because I had her trust, and the trust of the other group members. The room arrangement might not be reliable, but *I* was reliable. Also, I knew how to communicate with each child, and I knew to explain the changes in advance. I saw the potential for confusion and addressed it before it was a problem.

When she came into the group room, do you think I was true to my word? You bet I was. I was hyper-aware of the need to help each child find their seat. I embodied the role of the most gracious host at a party, the most attentive usher in a theater. My focus was solely on making sure everyone found their correct seat without emotional discomfort. I was like a marshaller on the airport runway who waves his light sticks to guide the jets to their gate. I even shushed a parent who tried to talk to me while all this took place! I had a mission at hand and I was going to see it through.

I am fully aware that not everyone is going to be as responsive as you and me. The world is full of those who cannot see the pain. Therefore, the more an Autistic child can communicate their perspective, or simply ask for help, the safer they will feel, and the safer they will be.

This is a simple example; the stakes do get much higher. What happens if a young adult is riding a public bus and the bus route changes? What if there is a misunderstanding and a child is suspended from school for being disrespectful to a teacher, when in fact that was not the child's intent at all? For these children, the potential social pitfalls are endless.

It is hard even for neurotypical people to stay calm and explain their point of view when under extreme stress. Imagine the life of an Autistic person. They might not have the ability to explain their emotional point of view even when they are calm. Therefore, learning to self-advocate is a long journey. Children often learn via play and friendships, but when friendships are lacking – as they are for so many children on the spectrum – then we have yet another urgent reason to make socialization accessible.

Play is the work of children. As a social coach you help your child with play, yes – but you also nurture small seeds to help your child grow toward social independence. Although we can't make it the world's goal to see the pain, you can make it *your* goal.

23

Planning a Successful Play Date

A play date gives your child the opportunity to form a one-on-one reciprocal relationship with another child, with all the subtle challenges that navigating friendships entails. How do you know if your child is ready? How do you know if *you* are ready? You'll know that both of you are ready when you have a good handle on things in your everyday life together.

Life does not have to be hunky-dory perfect before you consider planning a play date, but you do need to be able to make an honest assessment of your child's emotional and conceptual readiness. Reaching this point may feel like a journey of discovery – perhaps more of an adventure than you were anticipating. It can be messy. You will not have perfect clarity. Hopefully you have had some small breakthrough in the way that you interact with your child. You should feel you've claimed some new foothold of understanding, as shaky as it might be.

By contrast, if you started reading this book last Tuesday and have tried just a few accommodations with mixed results, then planning a play date is probably not going to help where more basic interventions haven't been given a proper chance for success. If nothing else has succeeded, then it's very doubtful that jumping into a play date is going to be the answer.

If you hurry, it hurts your child.

Every child is different, of course, and yours might be an exception. Let's do a reality check. Do you have accommodations in place for good communication? Have you implemented Family Fun Time in your schedule? Is it going well?

A successful play date is a big milestone, but it should come as a small step on a continuum, not a giant hurdle to jump over with no preparation. It's important not to give your child more social responsibility than they are ready to handle. This is not to limit their freedom, but to limit epic failures, which are not uncommon. You certainly don't want your child to be overwhelmed, discouraged, confused, or disoriented so that they never want to socialize again. Instead, build on the positive. Create a track record of success.

Do you have enough positive experiences to build on? That is when you and your child are ready for a play date.

Don't set your child up for failure. *Play date* includes the word "play." Play is supposed to be fun. It should leave a child wanting more. Will your child see it this way? If you can't say 'yes' with confidence, then identify the problem areas and look for accommodations that will help. Maybe this chapter will give you some ideas, but keep in mind that everything here is based on groundwork laid earlier. To plan a successful play date, you begin with everything you have accomplished so far, and then help your child take the next step toward independent social learning.

Help for your child comes with the next small success that is possible today. A play date should feel like a natural next step. Is your child ready? Are you ready?

Then let's begin.

Who Does the Planning?

You do, at least at first, even for older children and teenagers. Planning a get-together is a complex social activity, and if you start by expecting your child to pick up the phone and make it happen on their own, a successful outcome is unlikely. The very idea is emotionally overwhelming for many on the spectrum. Don't be discouraged, this is to be expected. The ability to independently plan a play date seems to be among the last areas to develop. Of course that's a generalization, but please keep it in mind. Autistic children can enjoy attending play dates long before they can initiate one on their own.

With help and guidance, your child will enjoy the events you plan for them. Then (we hope) each success will create motivation for them to plan independently.

What Are Your Child's Needs?

Where do you think your child needs the most help on a play date? You will have some idea from your Family Fun Time experience. Now you need to consider what might present difficulties when you expand beyond your own family.

An honest assessment is important, but can be emotionally difficult to do. For this reason I recommend having play dates with children who are also on the spectrum. The other parents should be doing the same assessment of their own child, and hopefully everyone involved will therefore be sensitive and supportive of each other. Remember, your child has strengths, too, and these will come into focus when you do an assessment. Here are some general questions to consider:

Play Date Social Assessment

- ☐ What are your child's interests?
- ☐ Should the play date cater to these interests or is your child willing to try different things?
- ☐ How does your child handle conflict with a friend?
- ☐ What are your child's concept gaps? How well do they "learn past" the gaps?
- ☐ How much social freedom is your child ready to accept?
- ☐ What accommodations are necessary?
- ☐ How well does your child problem solve? Can they do it independently?
- ☐ Can your child negotiate appropriately with a friend?
- ☐ How does your child respond to not getting their way?
- ☐ Can your child self-advocate at the appropriate level for the social situation?
- ☐ How long can your child socialize independently without help?
- ☐ Can your child follow directions from the other parent?
- ☐ Are there safety concerns?

Think about the kind of support your child will need, especially at someone else's house. Do you need to be present at the play date? If so, in what capacity? At this point, we are looking at your child's areas of need. It is more comfortable to look at strengths, but a sincere assessment of vulnerable areas will allow you to support your child and help move things forward socially. The following are just a few examples. I encourage you to come up with your own list.

Self-Advocacy and Emotional Regulation
- ☐ Too nervous to ask for help
- ☐ Uncomfortable talking to other family members
- ☐ Uncomfortable with any change in routine
- ☐ Afraid of pets, thunderstorms, etc.
- ☐ Easily frustrated by losing a game
- ☐ Becomes over-stimulated and needs a break
- ☐ Has trouble getting words out in new situations
- ☐ Has behaviors which make others uncomfortable
- ☐ Voice volume is inappropriate for the environment
- ☐ Has meltdowns

Safety
- ☐ Will not stay in designated play areas
- ☐ Opens doors without knocking
- ☐ Is at risk for being bullied
- ☐ Is gullible or easily misled; might follow inappropriate suggestions
- ☐ Does not always know when or how to ask for help
- ☐ Cannot distinguish a small problem from an emergency

Social Vulnerability
- ☐ Needs help understanding personal space
- ☐ May touch other people's things without asking

- ☐ Is very impulsive
- ☐ Sensitive about apparent fairness
- ☐ Requires clear logical explanations
- ☐ Rigid about rules to games
- ☐ Does not distinguish mean teasing from friendly teasing
- ☐ Does not use the bathroom independently
- ☐ Has trouble understanding and giving compliments

You don't necessarily need to tell the other family every detail about your child's social assessment; it depends on how well you know the other family and how much you trust them. You do want to have a plan to maximize social success. Certainly you'll want to have some well-tested accommodations in mind for any difficult situations that are likely to come up.

Friendship Matching

Who should you invite to the play date? You (not your child) will need to take the lead, even if your child is of an age when children typically plan these things on their own. Simply asking your child who they would like to invite can have mixed results. They might not know who they want to play with. Or they may have an idea, but you know that it just won't work out. You don't just randomly ask someone to come over to your house if you have never talked to them before; an Autistic child might not be aware of this.

Your involvement might feel natural when planning for younger children, but it is a little unusual for the mother of a fifteen year old to call the parent of another teen for a play date. However, it is often necessary. You can see why starting with another child who is also on the spectrum can be more comfortable for everyone. It is best to start with another child who is equally invested in the fledgling relationship. Things are then more balanced. The parents pave the way, and the children will be more or less equally in need of help.

Ideally your child will be involved in a social group with opportunities to meet potential friends. It may be a small group for Autistic children, or a larger community group such as a library program.

> **Mutual Support**
>
> The more compassionate and understanding the parents are of each other's children, the more successful the play date will be. You and the other parents can plan together, share accommodations that work for each child, and give the new friendship the best chance for success. Mainly, you want the children to feel good about themselves. In the beginning, they will surely need parental guidance. We want to keep them motivated to socialize again.
>
> How will other parents interact with your child? You can't expect them to know the best interaction style. They might be great at it, or maybe not. It is certainly easier when parents get along and are nonjudgmental of each other's children.
>
> Thinking about the whole play date process from beginning to end is the key to success, and involvement of other motivated parents brings mutual support.

I run social accessibility groups, and I put a great deal of attention on group composition to assure that participants are compatible on many levels. This does not always translate into a match for play dates (friendship matching is but one of my goals), though of course I am always on the lookout for potential matches. I have often seen children miss the friendship overtures of someone else in their group. They have no idea that someone is trying to be their friend. Fortunately, a professional is present to help clarify the situation. This is a very exciting time for everyone. Finding someone who wants to be a friend is an indescribably positive feeling.

Although your child can meet potential friends nearly anywhere, most organizations do not have the resources or expertise to help with friendship matching for children on the autism spectrum, so I'll give you an idea of how I do it. It's a role you might need to play as you encounter potential friends for your child.

If I see that some group members have the potential to be friends, I start to plant seeds in a slow but steady way. I talk about things they have in common and emphasize similar activities that they have both done in the past, such as bowling or miniature golf. I might even learn if they have gone to the same bowling alley before. This paves the way for a possible play date.

After I know the group members get along fairly well, I ask them if they would ever like to get together outside of group. The younger children will often beat me to the punch and start asking each other to come to their house. Older children and teens are typically much more hesitant, and my first suggestion of a get-together might be met with silence. The whole idea is initially just too overwhelming.

I breeze right past it and change the subject.

Then something interesting happens: each child starts to believe that the other might really want to be their friend. If I have done my job then they trust me to help with the process. This is why I encourage parents to prove their value as an ally and a social coach: these children need someone with skills and guidance they can trust to help them on their challenging adventure.

Now we are ready to move forward, but it still takes some time. The parents need to get involved. In the waiting room I encourage group members to mention their desire to get together so that their parents will rise to the challenge. Some parents are thrilled with the idea, while others are more reluctant. I believe some of the reluctant ones just don't want to endure rejection yet again. They may be burned out or self-conscious about their child's behavior. They might not have the energy; perhaps they're not comfortable with the other parents. I also have another theory: some are so accustomed to their child not having play dates that the family schedule never needed to include time for it. It does take time to plan and pull off a successful play date; it doesn't happen on its own.

I would love it if more organizations were able to take the lead with this important work. You may need to take the lead yourself in the social groups your child participates in.

Building the Concept

Not everyone will have a professional to do the groundwork, so let's take a closer look at how to do it yourself. Don't just jump to asking a potential friend to come over to the house. You need to set up the idea as much as you can because the children involved might not initially be into it. It can be too much of a shock to their system.

The Connection Formula

Suppose there is someone in your child's after school games club who you think would be a good friend for your child. Let's call him Brent. You have seen your child play Go Fish with Brent, and signs are good that this would be a successful activity for them to try outside of school. You've had the opportunity to chat with Brent's mother, and feel comfortable asking for a play date. Now it's time to bring your child on board.

Introduce the idea very gradually. Your child has never seen Brent outside of school. Is there a concept gap here, one that would cause confusion when the line between people he sees at home and at school begins to blur? It's hard to anticipate what the reaction will be. Did you ever run into someone outside the setting where you normally see them? (It can be mildly disorienting to spot your doctor in the supermarket.) An Autistic child might take it in stride, have an extreme reaction, or fall anywhere in between. Let's be sure that your child is well prepared.

Start by planting some seeds. For example, while playing Go Fish at home, casually mention that you noticed Brent likes playing the game, too. Then you might add that Brent's mom likes the game as well. Paint the image that Brent and his mom play Go Fish at their house, just like we are doing now. It creates an image of Brent in a different environment. It is also showing Brent's mom in a different way. The gist of your message is this:

👍 *Brent and his mom have fun at home just like us, and they enjoy some of the same things we do.*

This gives a concrete way for your child to imagine Brent and his family outside of the school setting.

Depending on your child's interest you can have fun with the topic and add something like this:

👍 *I wonder if they play at their kitchen table like we are. Hmm, I wonder if they even have a kitchen table. Not everyone has a table in the kitchen. Some people have a counter and some people have no place to eat in the kitchen. I seriously doubt that they play on the kitchen floor!*

There's no need to look for any particular response here. Just keep playing the game.

Talking to your child about Brent's family and using a common experience such as a card game is a good way to build a bridge of social understanding. This is helpful because it is a specific idea that can be used to manifest the play date in the future – a way of making a future get-together less abstract. Building the concept this way gives a much greater chance for success than simply asking, "Would you like to invite Brent over to our house, yes or no?" If you haven't planted the right seeds, then the answer might be "no," stopping the idea in its tracks.

Even if the answer is "yes," you can't assume things will go smoothly. When Brent arrives and actually knocks on the door it could be a jolt to your child. It might feel like social overload – too many new social experiences and feelings happening too quickly. If there has not been enough preparation, the play date experience could be a case of too much too quickly. Set up the idea in advance and try to anticipate the potential bumps in the road. Take your time and plant the right seeds.

Preparing Your Child for the Play Date

A play date is much like Family Fun Time, but there are a number of special considerations.

Structure and Backup Plans

As usual, you will want some well-planned activities, and lots of backup plans. On the other hand, the play date can be somewhat less structured than Family Fun Time. This is just as well, because it's simply not practical for two families to devise a detailed plan that will exactly match the needs of both children. To some extent you'll need to let them have the experience that they're going to have, although adults should be ready with those backup plans. Our hope is that your child is now ready to handle a little more social freedom. You do not need to look for perfection, just something that does not feel like failure to your child. Based on the outcome, you will learn and adjust in future play dates.

Visual Guides

Another key difference is location: the play date is not necessarily held at home. Even when it is, one of the children will be in an unfamiliar place. How will they cope with this? What sort of information do you suppose is needed? This is something to discuss in advance with the other parent, as each child may require different levels of structure and support.

The hosting parent should provide a visual guide that incorporates pictures of family members who will be there, pets, and the home itself if possible, including the door where guests will enter. A picture of the activity room and even the location of the bathroom can be helpful. Will there be snacks in the kitchen? Then include a snapshot of this area, too. Make the unfamiliar familiar. Clearly this works best for a child who is already used to picture guides.

Rule Variations

There is one more important consideration that makes a play date different from Family Fun Time: different families might use different rule variations. Ideally parents will choose activities that both children are already familiar with, especially for the first play dates. If different game rules will be used, explain them.

> 👍 *Did anyone ever tell you that the rules of Go Fish change in different places? Our family uses the matching pair rule, not the four-of-a-kind rule...*

It's obviously best to settle the question of rule variations in advance by discussing the planned activities with the other parent. If you'll be using different rules, try them out during Family Fun Time to uncover any negative reactions before the play date.

Sequential Walkthrough

Consider doing a sequential walkthrough in advance of the get-together to review the main parts of the plan with your child.

Who will lead the activities? How will I know what to do? Your child might not ask such questions, but it's a good idea to bring some accommodations into play (the 1-5 safety scale, for example) to uncover any anxiety and alleviate any worry they may have. Children might need to know anything from what snacks will be served to how to ask permission to use the bathroom. Don't give unnecessary details; give information based on what you already know about your child's sensitivities, needs and concerns.

In any discussion of the play date, try to be light and conversational. There is no need for a lecture. For your child this should not be like cramming for a test. Make it a natural extension of the sort of activities they have already engaged in and enjoyed. If you feel like you are overwhelming your child by putting lots of attention on the upcoming play date, then quickly dial back the barrage of information and just plan to participate more directly when the day arrives. On the other hand, if your child has lots of questions, do your best to answer.

During the Play Date

The day is here. The children are as ready as they're going to be. What happens now?

Tour of the Home

It's a good idea to start with a tour of the home – at least the parts that are relevant. Explain what rooms the children can enter and what is off limits. For example, you don't want a teenage boy to enter the sister's bedroom unannounced. Show where the bathroom is, and mention to knock before entering if you feel that might be necessary. Do not assume visitors will know how to do this.

Household Procedures

Let the visiting child know there may be different procedures for household activities such as getting a snack in the kitchen. Some children help themselves and act too familiar in another person's home. Others need permission to start eating their snack, or might not be comfortable asking for more. Hopefully any real concerns will have been identified in advance, but don't expect a child to memorize all the procedures.

The Connection Formula

Parent Participation

Should both parents be present during the play date? Should one of you lead the activities? This depends on many factors such as the age of the children, their developmental level, and the mutual comfort of the two families. In some cases I recommend that the parents participate in the activities. This is appropriate even for teenagers when the support is needed. At the very least, a parent needs to be nearby for key transitions or to resolve problems if any arise.

Remember, we don't want to set these children up for failure by giving them more social responsibility than they can handle. If you lead the activities, you can draw on your own Family Fun Time experience, but you'll want to make things a little less choreographed because you probably won't know the other child well enough.

Rule Review

Hopefully you've already prepared your child for any rule variations. A reminder is prudent at the beginning of a game, and guidance during the game can be necessary as well. It's important to plan details like this, even if it seems like over-planning. I have seen children become uncomfortable not only when they did not understand the rules, but also when another participant was unclear about the rules. It's as if they are playing different games. In fact, there's no *as if* about it. When the rules are not clear to everyone, they *are* playing different games. Now *that* can be confusing! Without some effective self-advocacy skills, this is a very awkward social situation for children on the spectrum to resolve on their own.

* * *

It's easy to believe this level of detailed planning isn't needed for your child, and maybe you're right. But are you really *really* sure? Are you willing to risk your child's self-confidence by leaving anything to chance?

The Schedule

Do you need a specific activities schedule? You should know the answer based on your Family Fun Time experience. Usually a written schedule is necessary for a child's first few play dates.

I recommend short get-togethers in the beginning. It is always best to leave the children wanting more. Here's an example of a short agenda (about 45 minutes) that you could show to the children:

- ☐ Start time: between 4:00-4:15
- ☐ Tour of house
  Parents show which rooms we can go in
- ☐ Introductions
  (List family members who will be there)
- ☐ Play Go Fish in the family room
  Parents will review the rules
- ☐ Snack at the table in the kitchen
  Snack is fruit and juice
- ☐ Trivia Game (if time)
  A parent will run the game
- ☐ Goodbye
- ☐ End time: between 4:45-5:00pm

It's important to keep track of time and give updates if the schedule needs to be modified. If parents aren't leading the activities, one may need to jump in when it's time for a transition. The introduction of activities is important, and transitions from one activity to another need to be as clear as possible. You can see the similarity to Family Fun Time. The structure can be somewhat more relaxed, but at key moments a parent will be necessary. In particular, don't expect the other parent to know what is going to be hard for your child.

Eventually, the adults may be able to fade into the background as the children do some activities together, then jump back in and help out as needed. You'll discover a rhythm: fade into the background, jump in and participate, fade into the background again.

Let Fun Bubble to the Top

Because children on the autism spectrum probably have not socialized successfully as much as their neurotypical peers, there will be gaps in their social development. The older the child, the greater the gaps can be. If your child has never had true friends and now starts to socialize at age sixteen and is happy, then that is fantastic! Just keep in mind the many social experiences that your child has missed. Involvement in community social events such as scouts or soccer does not necessarily mean your child has suddenly caught up and learned to socialize. If these activities bring enjoyment, that alone is pretty great, but it is not the same as developing a true friendship. Family Fun Time is a path to play dates, and play dates are a path to friendships, especially when both children are invested in the goal.

Until you get some experience with play dates, you won't know exactly what will be needed when you bring another child into the picture. In my work, I never know what will be needed for a particular child until I get to know them, so I plan for every contingency I can think of. I have a complete structure in place, with many accommodations at my fingertips. I call it a *flexible structure* because I am always changing it as I see what is, and is not, needed. As I've mentioned, it's easier to start with a structure and relax it later than it is to create one from nothing in the moment. Now of course you have a big advantage over me: you already know your child. The play date involves another child, so ideally the parents plan together.

A good social coach is confident in the game plan, so think about the social choreography of the play date to the point where you feel confident. As you (and your child) gain experience, then it is okay to become more relaxed with the plan.

A flexible structure lets fun bubble to the top.

24

Safe Passage

If social independence came naturally to you when you were young, then today you probably don't even need think about it. On the other hand, for someone on the autism spectrum, socializing and social independence do not come naturally at all. I've met many adults on the spectrum who are challenged by this very thing on a daily basis. I primarily work with children, but I am always thinking about their future. I imagine what they will be like when they grow up. Have I offered them enough support, tools, and confidence to maximize their quality of life as adults? Getting by is not enough. I want them to thrive. I know you do too.

The Connection Formula is about changing the way you interact with your child, but it is more than that. It is about changing the way you perceive your child's world. That is the key and, for many, the stumbling block that stops the process before it begins.

It would be nice to start with empathy, drawing on our own emotional experiences to understand what it feels like to be continuously misunderstood. If empathy opens your heart and gives you a measure of patience, then it's a good place to begin. But there's a catch. Empathy has to do with recognizing and sharing feelings that someone else is experiencing. But how can you feel empathy without a true understanding of how your child experiences life? Can you empathize with emotions when you have no idea what they are?

The world of emotions is a very deep place. If you haven't experienced confusion at a fundamental level, then you need to stretch your imagination in order to have some inkling of what it is like for your child. You need to be a patient detective to discover what might be going on beneath the surface. I have seen people make bad situations worse by assuming they know what is going on in a child's mind when they couldn't be more wrong. It's terribly easy to believe that your basic assumptions about human interaction and behavior hold true for everyone, and that's the catch with empathy. It's a sympathetic impulse that says, "Oh, I know just how you feel." But in reality, you don't.

It's best to admit that you don't know. Some parents who come to me already have. This may leave them with a feeling of desperation, but it's actually a move in the right direction. Giving up your preconceptions is a good thing. You still have compassion, and compassion means you want to help. You have begun to autism-ize your thinking. How do you take it further?

Think of your own need to feel safe and understood. If nothing else, this will motivate you to consider what life might be like for an Autistic child trying to protect themselves when the world becomes a confusing and scary place. Are you with me so far? If you can take it on faith – or perhaps sense, even a little, the gargantuan nature of a child's inner struggle – then you are on the right track.

You have put your toe in the ocean.

Now I invite you to go a little deeper. Consider that some Autistic children *never* feel safe and understood. For them the world has always been a source of confusion, insecurity, and yes, even imminent danger. This may be hard to imagine, but I assure you it is sometimes the case. For such a child, life can be an incredibly frightening battleground in a nonstop struggle for emotional survival. And this is where our journey began, with the idea that such a struggle could be taking place right before your eyes, and you simply would not know.

But let's go deeper still, because there is light at the end of this tunnel.

Parents don't want to believe that someone they love could be enduring such a burden, but the struggle is not part of autism per se; it comes largely from the outside, at the borders of our inaccessible neurotypical world. So here is the most important thing for you to understand: When you allow yourself to imagine what an Autistic child's life just might feel like from the inside, then your compassion will have something to connect to. You will begin to see behind the curtain, and the possibilities expand accordingly. Once you maximize communication and minimize the fear – in other words, when you make life accessible – you may be encouraged, even delighted, by what you find.

If an Autistic child's struggle is greater than many believe, so too is the expansiveness of their viewpoint, the depth of their experience, and the richness of what they have to offer as you get to know their world.

* * *

What further advice can I give? I've shown you the compassion gap; I don't doubt you feel compassion. I've offered accommodations to make socialization accessible to a child with a social learning disability. Just as we remove barriers to mobility for people with a physical disability, we wish to remove barriers to an Autistic child's sense of safety and connection. If I've sensitized you to some of those barriers, then we have a great start.

Now you have the tools you need to connect with a child on the autism spectrum. Yet the tools alone are not enough, and I hope I've made that clear. Seeing the need for accommodations is even more important than the accommodations themselves. Why? Because if you understand the reason for them you can then create your own. You will see life from your child's perspective, and you'll be able to adapt your parenting style to convey social information in a way that is meaningful to them.

Remember that this is as much about attitude and demeanor as about any particular technique. Accommodations come from a sincere desire to connect. Use them in a calm and comforting manner. Be gentle and direct. Bring the lightest touch you can. Believe in the possibilities. Autism-ize your thinking and watch the relationship with your child blossom and grow. Not only will your child feel safe and understood, *you* will feel understood by your child. Connecting at this level is a win-win situation. Both parent and child are happier.

I realize there is a tremendous amount of information to absorb. It's not reasonable to expect anyone to incorporate it all at once. Start with one accommodation and build from there. Don't feel you need to rush. Removing one barrier at a time *does* make a difference, and incremental changes will usually be easier for your child. The larger goal is to keep using your creative imagination to find the many ways to connect to your child's world, help them connect to yours, and so become your child's lifeline. It's an ongoing journey that is never really done. But, then again, you're never done being a parent, are you?

This book is a call to creativity. I hope I've inspired you to try a few new ideas. Will the children we work with today have safe passage as adults in this topsy-turvy neurotypical world – a world that clearly has much to learn about autism?

With your help this will be a reality.

Made in the USA
Lexington, KY
17 April 2015